The Silent Sanctuary

—— TOME I ——

Prânâyâma & Meditation

Patrice Godart

DISCLAIMER

The author and the publisher are not responsible for any injury resulting from the practice of instructions included in this book. The described activities, physical or other, could be tiresome or dangerous for certain individuals and so the reader should consult a medical professional beforehand.

Discovery Publisher

French Edition, 2022, © Patrice Godart, Discovery Publisher
All rights reserved.

English Edition, 2025, @ Discovery Publisher
All rights reserved.

Author: Patrice Godart
Translator: Steve Cannon

Cover Artwork © Discovery Publisher

Title: *The Silent Sanctuary: Prânâyâma and Meditation* / Patrice Godart

Subjects: Yoga | Mind-Body Relations | Metaphysical

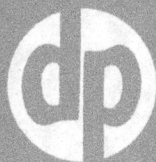

616 Corporate Way
Valley Cottage, New York
www.discoverypublisher.com
editors@discoverypublisher.com

New York • Paris • Dublin • Tokyo • Hong Kong

Table of Contents

The Silent Sanctuary

— TOME I —

Prânâyâma & Meditation

Patrice Godart

The Silent Sanctuary aims to present a vast panorama of representations and practical methods, essentially Tantric, leading to meditation and altered states of consciousness and energy.

✧

This volume is the first part and deals more specifically with breathing techniques and the manipulation of prâna through subtle or psychic breathing exercises for meditation.

✧

The Silent Sanctuary is also an attempt to bridge the gap between Sri Aurobindo's thought, the practice of traditional Indian yogas and life on the outside.

✧

The section on self-knowledge is inspired by the thinking of Sri Aurobindo and The Mother. Some of these representations have already been explored in our previous books.

✧

The practical part is directly indebted to the personal teachings of Paramahansa Satyananda Saraswati and other Indian teachers.

We would like to pay special tribute
to Gangadhar † for the original
engraving on pages 15, 130,
and all the faces of the kriyâs.

✳

Our thanks to Béatrice Savignac
for the illustrations on pages 61 and 62,
Marie Duvollet for the illustrations
pages 87, 96, 164, 190, and all the
web designers and practitioners
who made their drawings and photos
available to all.

✳

In the practical part, we have tried to establish as
many relationships as possible between the chapters.
This makes it possible to study each chapter much
more independently.

✳

We have had to retain a number of Sanskrit
terms and use a few specific ones. Readers will
find a glossary on the following page and at
the end of the book.

✳

Quotes from Sri Aurobindo and The Mother
are published with the kind permission of Sri
Aurobindo Ashram Trust Pondicherry, India.

INTRODUCTION

Silence is not absence, emptiness or nothingness. Silence vibrates within us and lives at the heart of every element in the universe. This silence is not the opposite of speech or noise; it is a state, a substance, a prime condition that exists outside time and would continue to exist even if the physical universe were to disappear.

To experience this silence is to discover an extraordinary inner existence and fullness. It can be expressed in different ways for each individual, but vibration, life, light and bliss are the most natural expression of prâna practices.

Today's homo *sapiens* knows only the extension of his own egocentric and superficial reference points; he ignores that there is also a depth, and that it is from this depth that the world is created at every moment. The surface world cannot create; it can only reproduce and rearrange the same elements in new combinations. And even then, the variety of these combinations remains limited to its representations, which today are stubbornly rationalist and materialistic.

In every age and every tradition, there have been people who have discovered this depth within themselves, but in penetrating this vast silence, they have often turned away from the world of the surface and appearance, leaving it to turn in on itself and perpetuate its illusions, impasses and suffering.

For we can enter this inner silence and explore its riches by leaving life, but we can also enter this silence and return to the center of a cornucopia to heal ourselves and transform our nature, but also our environment and our world. That's what we've chosen to do.

We spend our lives trying to make a place for ourselves in the sun, but in the depths of our being we discover an existence in ourselves beside which the quest for existence in the world is no more than a narrow, clumsy attempt.

We seek intense sensations and multiply our activities, but isn't wanting to live intensely actually seeking intense vigilance? In interiorization, we discover a vigilance within ourselves, natural, unsupported, independent and limitless.

We chase after pleasures, consumer goods and the tools of power that our technology offers us, but at the heart of this silence lies a plenitude that intoxicates us deliciously, and the source of a power that fascinates and moves us.

Living under stress is nothing if there's a good reason for it. But it's unbearable to build your life on a lack of meaning and emptiness that generates chronic anxiety.

Yoga, and in particular Indian yoga, which is still somewhat resistant to the invasion of technological globalization and has flourished in incredible diversity for millennia right up to the present day, reminds us of this inner dimension at the heart of man and the world. It is from this depth that humanity has drawn all its richness. For in truth, the world is upside down, and all we know of life is its bark.

However, the yoga we know has further reinforced this false image that we have to leave outer life to know the Truth. For in reality, this message contradicts our nature. All our energies are directed towards action, creation, organization and mastery of the world. Has Nature placed in us a program and an impulse contrary to the truth? Are we conditioned to nourish and live out the fantasies of our minds? Are we condemned to receive the crumbs from Life's table, mixed with a few poisoned seeds? If so, then Nature would be provocative and malevolent, our mind would be our enemy, and life would be nothing but a gigantic hoax!

So why enter into the depths of ourselves if it's only to achieve immobility and inaction, and destroy the life energy that sustains us?

It's here that we can fully appreciate the secrets Sri Aurobindo has rediscovered.

The first secret is that the self we know is only the most superficial part of a vaster, deeper, *subliminal* nature, close to eternal truths and rich in

multiple potentialities and qualities of which we know only a pale reflection in our surface nature. We are not just a collection of difficulties
and imperfections, irreducibly subject to dualities and egocentricity. Our
mind is much larger than we suppose. It extends deep inside ourselves
and rises into higher and higher layers, conscious, vast, luminous, full
of bliss, working faster and faster up to a new mode of knowledge, by
identity. This is where our consciousness of division, suffering and evil, is
entirely replaced by a vision of unity which, at its peak, can be transfigured into a *supramental* consciousness, as Sri Aurobindo calls it, capable
of fertilizing unity and multiplicity into each other and giving birth to a
new man and a new Earth. The mind we use places us on the first step of
knowledge. Great Nature expects us to climb the next.

The second secret is that we harbor within us a *spiritual individuality*, which Sri Aurobindo calls *the Psychic Being* and others call *the Soul*,
whose raison d'être is to perfect man, in a progressive evolution through
multiple lives, to make him conscious and reunite him with his origin
of perfection and infinitude. We have been told so often that perfection
is not of this world, and that Truth, wholeness or harmony can only be
found outside human nature and life! This essential individuality is a cornucopia, a link between the all possibility of the eternal, infinite Cosmic
Spirit and the unlimited perfection of universal Nature. Indian tradition
calls it Chaïtya Purusha, the Conscious Being. And to bring Him even
closer to us, He creates three emanations of Himself, one in each of the
three parts of our nature – mental, vital and physical – which nourish and
support a profound nature we know nothing about, and which holds
unsuspected resources of consciousness and power that we could really
use. We can decree that it's not possible for this to exist, but we can also
set out to experience it. Then we'll quickly realize whether it's myth or
reality.

The third secret reveals the stratagem of *Mâyâ*, the Cosmic Illusion. It's
the discovery that this powerful silence within ourselves and the world
reveals itself in the aspect in which we approach it: static and unchanging, in the aspect of out-of-this-world *consciousness*, or dynamic and
evolving in the form of omnipresent *energy* and conscious *force*. So, if
we so wish, we have the power and awareness we need to accompany our

daily lives and drive our evolution.

So there is a bliss and a joy, an awareness, a peace, a light, a knowledge, a power, that either distances us from life and the world **or** perfects, transfigures and fulfills Nature and life. *It all depends on our intention and representation*. We've been given a free will that's hard to manage, and we have all the philosophies to affirm both Truth and its opposites, but isn't it worth the effort if we can become the actors of our own perfection?

Apart from the ancient Vedas, these secrets have only recently been explored and applied to life by a handful of beings. They are given to us so that we ourselves can become the creators and conquerors of a flourishing nature and a transfigured Earth.

We've been mystified by so many centuries of ignorance, unaware that half-knowledge is even greater ignorance, for it is a light that infallibly guides us into the error and misery of a life truncated by half, even if it is luminous. *"By a golden mask is covered the face of Truth"* says the Isha Upanishad. Today, we wake up with an inner fire, but soon we won't have the excuse of ignorance and innocence.

Today's Indian yogas express these two sides of Truth, one directed towards Consciousness, as in Vedanta or Buddhism, and the other towards spiritual energy and force, in Tantra. But they turned their backs on each other after losing the essence of the Vedic tradition, in which Truth encompassed both spheres of existence: higher and lower, Spirit and Matter. Even Indian Tantra today withdraws from human life rather than using its vast powers to transform it. And in this sense, the complete awakening of the spiritual power within man, *Kundalinî Shakti,* as well as the realization of the *Atman*, the universal Divine, by the great yogis of this century, who turn the tantric or yogi into a "living liberated one", *Jivanmukti,* are in fact only the first stage of spiritual realization, not its finality. For we are no longer talking about exclusively spiritual realization, but spiritual and material, individual and collective. An integral realization, as Sri Aurobindo puts it.

This is why the yogas of today's India have only half of the truth at their disposal. The other half is the frantic and futile search for truth by Western rationalism and productivism. The search for truth in the West and East are the two heads of the sphinx, representing unity and multiplicity, depth and surface, and they turn away from each other.

And what Sri Aurobindo expresses becomes so obvious when we have assimilated a little of these two very different worlds of Western life and Eastern philosophy! We're at a crucial point in human history when we need to reunite what we've separated, and rediscover the global vision and fullness of life, if we're to survive this impasse we're in. Thought based on division, even if embodied by the authority of Science, cannot lead to harmony and truth. On the contrary, we observe that the more technology develops and knowledge of matter becomes plethoric, the more life shrinks and the more human beings suffocate and degenerate.

And in the same way, a thought, however luminous, yogic and spiritual, that turns away from the Earth, cannot transform earthly life. We are faced with a double failure.

If we aspire to an integral truth, we must break out of the hypnotism that enslaves us to one or other of these two antagonistic yet complementary representations. But it is the yogas of India that can provide us with the method of our liberation, as well as a wide variety of tools for cultivating our inner garden and reconnecting with the silence of our soul **and** the soul of the world. Because the real method and the real resource lie within.

Fortunately, we don't have to create this silence out of thin air through our own efforts; we simply have to discover it within ourselves, and make our way towards it. Because that's what it's all about. When we discover within ourselves this silent substance, these spaces of freedom, this gaze that crosses or flies over, this self-sufficient happiness, this state of abundance in all the compartments of our psyche, we see that all this is within us and that it has always been there.

But for the person whose life is bitter or arid, and who discovers in meditation only the struggle against himself or herself, the litany of thoughts and the tyranny of emotions, more powerful because we have taken off our armor – or even sleep and the pains of the body, this can only be incomprehension or even, perhaps, provocation.

Meditation is a difficult art, as it is for any newcomer to any profession, and even more so here, because we've come face to face with a virgin forest that we've always ignored.

So we must persevere, learn the difficult lesson of self-acceptance, muster our aspiration, confidence and sincerity to soothe the mind and gradually open a passageway to the inner self. For this, we need to rediscover a sense of discipline, adopt a realistic progression and choose an effective method.

Why is meditation so difficult if we are naturally this deep self, one with the universe, and if we have all these resources within us? Because we've been taught to identify ourselves not with this essential self, but with a representation, an image of our individuality that has been imposed on us by our environment, our upbringing and our personal history, the ego.

And this is surely the main reason why it takes us so much time, so much effort and exercise, and so much inventiveness: to take that little self by surprise or to persuade it to let go and step aside.

Indeed, what would become of us without our efforts and pains, without the thickness of our toil, without our fears and hopes, without the thrusts of our will, the cohort of our desires and the constructs of our minds? We probably prefer to have the impression of controlling and directing our lives and our environment in our own way, even if the result remains limited. Rather, perhaps, live mediocrely, and feel free, than live better, but under external influence?

Otherwise, we'd be able to reunite and reconcile the surface world and the world within in no time, just as we naturally could when we were still a young child.

On the other hand, we lack maturity. Everything in our lives bears witness to the youthful defects of our conscience. We lack awareness, we lack real strength, and our faith in life and in ourselves is limited and fragile. In a word, we lack *consciousness-strength*, *shakti* as we say in India.

In this way, we've put our finger on the two resistances or obstacles that stand in the way of our natural evolutionary program: the ego and the lack of consciousness-strength.

But it's precisely to nourish this inner existence, to awaken our inner strength and intensify and elevate our inner gaze that we must touch this static yet dynamic silence within us, and regenerate ourselves there.

We need strength and maturity more than ecstasy. Above all, we need peace, structure, balance and discernment if we are to bring more intensity, light, grandeur and diversity into ourselves. Life is too vast, Nature is too big, reality is both too complex and too simple, for Truth can only be wholeness and infinite bliss.

So it's not easy to let ourselves be imbued with this silent vibration, even though it's the shortest route to fulfilling the human being we dream of being, and to seeing him or her grow naturally towards what we call the ideal or divinity, which is nothing other than the width, the light, the perfection we must become, and the reunification with our center, which is also, quite naturally, the same center in everyone and everything.

Yoga, then, is not only an excellent method of relaxation for our bodies and minds, nor the difficult art of diving into ourselves; it is also a culture of the true, the vast, the beautiful, the consciousness that expands and refines, the intelligence that resolves and the strength that heals and transforms. It's also a world of creativity and subtlety, a science of consciousness and being in contrast to the science we know, which explores energy and feeds the self and the ego.

The third millennium is upon us. It won't be an exclusive world of super-technology that will bring us more dreams and external power. We've already buried that dream, because we see that it leads to the alienation of our innermost selves and a disregard for the just and beneficial laws of life. This phony power actually builds our own fragility. Nor will it be a global economic superstructure that will further enrich a privileged few while increasing the material and moral misery of mankind, while plundering nature and infesting the Earth. It won't be.[1]

Firstly, because this model is a dead end that will lead humanity to complete degeneration or extinction. Secondly, because people are gradually waking up from the ignorance and unconsciousness in which they have been kept, and because they cannot always be mystified. This is the price we pay for the spread of means of communication and education. When consciousness grows, in a healthy environment, it becomes a beacon that

---

1. This preface, written over twenty years ago, named two dangers: the advent of transhumanism and a global financial hegemony cutting the world to shreds. Today, we see a completely different reality, with the advent of this totalitarian world government, which is using a virus as a biological weapon and a vaccine as an improved biological weapon, to achieve planetary genocide and the enslavement of all humanity, in parallel with the destruction of all spirituality, all culture, all differentiation, all traditions.

pierces the darkness of life and highlights all its imperfections and contradictions.

The third millennium will see the emergence of a conscious base and the revolt of Nature or Spirit that will force the dominant powers and nations, with the help of this base, to enter the mold of human unity, of a new vision of life, of truth, universality, fraternity, harmony and inner and outer beauty, within the framework of individual and collective evolution. For truth, if we want it to be whole, can only be evolutionary. It will be the union and fertilization of the two worlds of energy and consciousness, matter and spirit. The impasse in which humanity has locked itself, and the constant rise of individual consciousness, can only lead to a growth of consciousness in a world based on an integral truth of unity and multiplicity, in which all the elements of life must be represented. This is the challenge humanity must take up and succeed in.

Probably never before have so many ways of calming thought, achieving inner silence, transforming emotion, mastering our vitality and internal energy, accessing numerous altered states of consciousness and thus developing, expanding or elevating it, been brought together. This is both a formidable argument for convincing the mind that it's possible, and a particularly rich working tool that everyone can use as they wish and according to their nature. This may make our selection more difficult, as we are more accustomed to a one-sided, exclusive approach and simplistic recipes, but we deliberately want to encourage this integral vision and approach, which we consider indispensable.

We've been looking for a perspective on self-transformation that's neither exclusively mystical nor reserved for nature's privileged, well-born, well-endowed and flawless. If it's true that the spiritual dimension, containing all perfections, resides at the heart of the world and of man, then it must be the most natural thing in the world! And so there's no need to make a big deal of it and cover it in a cloak of impenetrable esotericism! We've been looking for a natural fulcrum, universally shared by human beings since they first looked up at the stars, based on need, on man's most essential needs, his existence, his individuality, his aspiration to rise and progress, his deepest eternal dreams.

We love Sri Aurobindo's constant concern for an integral vision, because we are totally convinced that truth can only be integral and therefore evolutionary, since we are limited. On the other hand, Nature has produced a human being of infinite diversity.

From all this stems the need for a multiplicity of methods and practices to serve this global self-transformation, as well as a multitude of paths. In a total vision, all paths become complementary, and any sectarianism is the mark not only of a limited vision, but also of a conscious desire to diminish the value of other paths, to reject them, or even to fight them. It's not our choices that are the problem, it's our exclusions! Then we'll be able to offer not one, but several resources to any difficulty, and several solutions to any problem.

In this way, we can discover an art of posture, âsana, of breath, prânâyâma, or of the various tantric meditation techniques, which are not only at the service of a life turned inward, but just as capable of transfiguring in the same way our outer life and our profession as human beings. Then we'll be able to rediscover those new ideas championed by Sri Aurobindo or The Mother: the complete transformation of the ego and of human nature, the union of inner and outer life, the emergence and radiance of the individual Divine, the development of the dynamic as well as the passive spiritual aspect, or the vision of the Divine in everything and as everything that exists. These are the first fundamental steps before moving on to the higher stages they describe. We don't claim to be a guide.

We believe in the need to recognize both unity and wholeness, as well as diversity and uniqueness, and as Westerners to explore new paths of development that reconcile inner and outer life. We wish to highlight other representations of meditation, such as centering or dynamic junction at the heart of active life, or other representations of the Divine, not very widespread in the West, such as the Universal Mother, consciousness-force, our deepest self, our original center or simply our future perfection, our evolutionary becoming.

Finally, as we have said, meditation will no longer be considered solely from a spiritual point of view outside the life of the world. We will include the art of mastering the material of our consciousness, our *citta*, the basic substance of our mind, thoughts and images, to achieve the mental silence that is the condition for our access to the higher mind and the

Supraconscious. And we will generalize this idea that we can gather new resources – and the higher mind is one of them – that we need so badly to survive this collective madness and rebuild ourselves legitimately and take part in rebuilding the world according to our most beautiful dreams.

The Silent Sanctuary cannot explore all the different aspects of these new facets of meditation without ending up with a thick, indigestible volume. That's why this volume will be devoted to breathing techniques. The next volume will focus on vibratory and psychological methods.

The Silent Sanctuary is an invitation to inner discipline, but also to the self-confidence and deep strength that are natural to us and so much needed to rediscover the true meaning of our lives and the essence of our being. It's not a program for three weeks or three months, but an undertaking of passion, research, exploration and discovery, the satisfaction of a lifetime, in the law of right self-fulfilment.

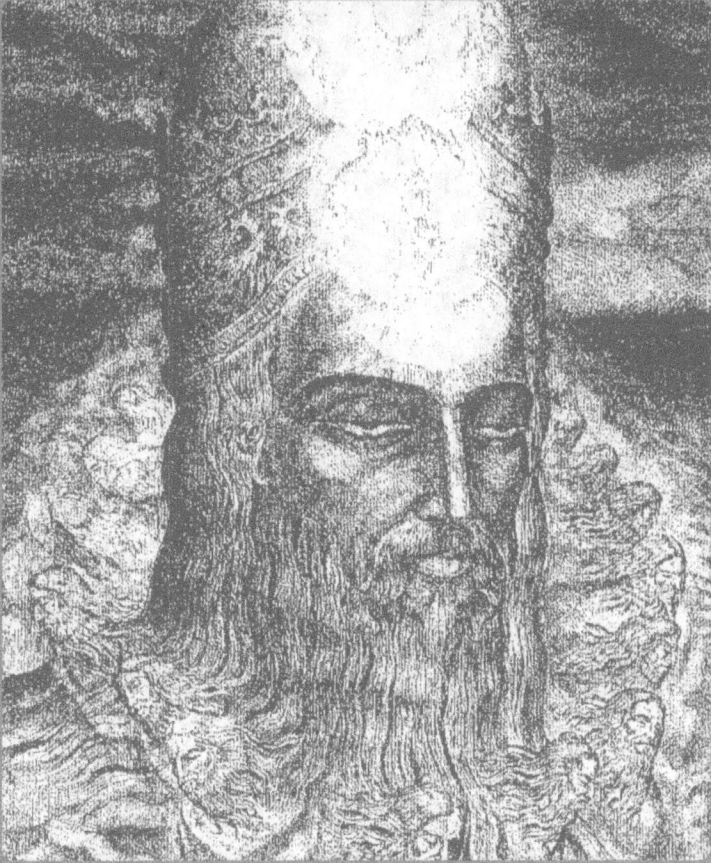
The Conscious Being, Purusha

I
A NEW APPROACH
TO MEDITATION

The unfinished man

Are we condemned to wander in our misery between the hopeless materialism of Science or economic liberalism, and the superficial morality of religion?

Our spiritual aspirations are not the product of religious conditioning, nor are our desires for human fulfillment the work of socio-cultural conditioning. Both are legitimate, stemming from the evolutionary program that has accompanied humanity since its birth. But they have been presented to us as antagonistic, and have been co-opted by the systems in place. So they leave us with a taste of bitterness and frustration, because they are two halves of the same fruit from the same seed.

Can we reconcile the bodily pleasure of running on a wet beach, the joy of the creator and the artist, the satisfaction of accomplishment of the entrepreneur, the passion of the philosopher, the researcher or the extreme sportsman, the bliss of the body, so intense that the slightest movement seems like lead, and the inner experience of an absolute existence in which the forms of the world appear empty and unreal to us, as if they were formed from the *papier-mâché* of theatrical sets? How can we reconcile the fullness of a conscious body, of a gesture overflowing with vital energy, the harmony of a true movement in a just action, the sensation of beauty, the devotion of the heart and the transcendent experience of the impersonal Absolute?

Is there a force capable of linking our human ideals with our spiritual aspirations? We dream so much of a fulfillment that is neither solely human nor exclusively spiritual, and of a coherence that embraces the whole of life!

Why meditate?

The Indian yoga tradition dates back several millennia. The Vedas, the Upanishads, the Agamas, the Puranas and the Tantras have today given rise to two major currents: Tantra and Vedanta.

According to Sri Aurobindo, in the earliest Vedic scriptures, the Divine was represented as everything that exists, whether invisible or visible, manifest or unmanifest. But later, in the era of the Upanishads, in striving to distinguish between the essential and the illusory, there was a split in Knowledge and a separation between the supreme Reality, Brahman, on the one hand, and Nature, perceived as an illusion, on the other. Vedanta[1], like Buddhism, followed this path, that of Consciousness.

At the same time, however, Tantra developed as a parallel movement, championing the divine energy, Shakti, of which Nature is a part. Vedantic yoga made *liberation* its exclusive goal, while Tantric yoga emphasized *liberation* and *enjoyment.* Sri Aurobindo, in his Integral Yoga, sees the need to integrate energy and consciousness into a wider vision, and prefers to speak of *liberation* and *transformation.*

The tantric path is less arduous, accepting the world and its pleasures, but within its priority of liberation. It should also be stressed that austerity and asceticism close the individual in on himself and isolate him, whereas enjoyment, the multiple pleasures of the senses, but also of all forms of prâna and consciousness, lead to the flowering of life and love. However, we must recognize that the extent of our success in this field will be proportional to our capacity for selfless enjoyment, for non-egotic involvement.

It's well established that spiritual liberation is the liberation from dualities and the ego. However, although the transformation of individual nature is recognized in Tantra, it is not an end in itself, nor is the transformation of the world, which includes all planes. Only Sri Aurobindo would place liberation and transformation on the same level, that of con-

1. The main current of yoga is Vedantic.

sciousness as well as energy and Nature, of both the individual and the world.

Vedanta seeks to attain the supreme Reality, *Sat-Chit-Ananda*, through consciousness, and therefore preferentially through meditation.

Tantra comprises two schools of philosophy and therefore two approaches, known as Left Hand Tantra and Right Hand Tantra. On the one hand, we have an insistence on the guru, the devata[1], the mantra and the yantra[2], and on the other, a complex and prolix set of techniques in the service of liberation by the individual Shakti, Kundalinî. But Tantric discipline also makes abundant use of the multiple relationships, which exist in every sense, between breath, prâna, citta[3] and the psyche. It's this latter practical approach that we'll be focusing on here.

As for Sri Aurobindo, in his Integral Yoga, he recommends relying on universal Shakti and the realization of the individual Divine, Jîvâtman – and its dynamic representation in the Heart, the Psychic Being.

For us, immersed and involved in the life of the world, at a time of violence, chaos, lies and selfishness, particularly in the spheres of power, which multiply resistance to the Good, to Knowledge and to true human progress, meditation, like other yogic practices, can no longer have the same meaning. We have seen the dangers of a spirituality that neglects the world, and has therefore refuted all truth[4]. And so it's only logical that today's world is falling apart, and that the exploitation of man and Nature, and human suffering, are everywhere on display. It's the end of a cycle of darkness, on the shore of another cycle of light. This new world bears the evidence of a truth that can only exist in wholeness. The individual and the collective, matter, Life, Mind, infinite and eternal Spirit. Nothing is lacking, and everything is moving towards its destiny of wholeness, consciousness as much as energy and therefore matter. This is Sri Aurobindo's vision.

---

1. Devata: deities, angels, divine presences and powers. The devata is characterized by its name (mantra) and symbol (yantra).

2. Yantra: form, symbol, mystical diagram, mandala.

3. Citta: The substance of consciousness.

4. The same is true of most of the religions and religious, philosophical and spiritual movements of the last two millennia – to put it briefly – which have distanced themselves from Nature, from matter, from integral Knowledge, from integral Truth. Each seeking truth outside of earthly life.

And with this in mind, we see the need for **liberation** and **transformation**. And because we live in a difficult world and self-transformation becomes so demanding, the acceptance of **enjoyment** in our lives becomes a resource. But it is not an end in itself, and merely accompanies the search for liberation and the transformation of our nature.

Enjoyment is everywhere, taking a thousand forms, and it happens to be a characteristic of Prâna, the energy of Life, both universal and individual. For Prâna awakens all the desires of the Universe and leads both to all the dualities responsible for our wanderings and suffering, and to energy, power and enjoyment. And the further we go along the Way, the more the principle of pleasure, joy and bliss is revealed, insofar as we don't exclude it.

Prâna brings enjoyment. The transformation of individual prâna brings bliss. We know the enjoyment of outer nature, which the body, mind and prâna gratify us with. But what do we know of the enjoyment of consciousness? Through breathing and meditation, through the combined growth and transformation of prâna and consciousness, we experience enjoyment and we honor and celebrate Life and journey along a less austere Path to self-realization.

This is how we come to emphasize three objectives in meditation:

◊ **Accessing the depths of consciousness and transcendence.**
◊ **Increasing our resources,** in a world where so-called progress is becoming hostile to the best in human beings and destructive of humanity's noble values.
◊ **To achieve mental silence** and thus mastery of thought and image. Because mental silence leads to our greatest resources, present and future, as well as to depth and transcendence.

This representation of meditation has another advantage: it prepares us for all forms of meditation, whatever the philosophies and spiritual currents, and this can be achieved in the midst of the modern world, however difficult it may be.

Transcendence

Here too, we distinguish between the transcendence of consciousness and the transcendence of nature.

The transcendence of consciousness is access to deep awareness, culminating in the experience of the Divine within, of the spiritual Self in the Deep Heart, the Psychic Being, and in the Supraconscious, which includes all mental planes higher than current human consciousness, towards the universal, towards eternal and infinite Consciousness in all its forms.

The Psychic Being[1] embodies both self-realization and transcendence. Note that in Maslow's pyramid of needs, these two concepts occupy the two highest degrees.

In the field of Nature, the need for transcendence covers all efforts to go beyond, to surpass oneself, to perfect oneself, to progress in all fields (perfecting a tool, a technique, an action, a psychological quality, a resource, a strategy, a field of knowledge...) Science, education and therapy have always been fields linked to the search for transcendence, but this is no longer true today, with the exception of a few isolated thinkers and researchers, often in opposition to the spirit of their discipline and their hierarchy.

The very meaning and driving force of evolution involves this impulse towards transcendence. It originates in the Vital Being, the part of the human being linked to Life, and its natural need for expansion, but also in the Higher Mind, at the origin, for example, of the need for knowledge and perfection. However, the strongest expression of transcendence and self-transcendence comes from the influence of the Psychic Being, as this is its most obvious characteristic.

Surpassing oneself in our society

Traditionally, as we have seen, meditation is associated with the search for transcendence of consciousness, spiritual realization, deep internalization and the training to acquire and cultivate this position of pure awareness, in opposition to the world of external energy and action. From this point of view, it is essentially a mystical, inner approach.

This objective is reinforced in our time by a model of civilization governed by scientific thought, subject to an exclusive rationalist and mate-

1. To avoid confusion between the words *psychic,* close to psychological, and *Psychic Being,* coming from a resolutely spiritual context, we capitalize the beginning of the word.

rialistic way of thinking, and subjugated to an economic world.

The influence of scientific thought in all fields is served by the impressive harvest of data describing matter and its workings. However, we must stress that this plethora of discoveries and knowledge is merely the description of a separating vision of Reality, truncated of its substance of unity and marked by the seal of incapacity of this dividing mind. We still know nothing of connected matter or connected life. This is evident not only in the limits and impasses of medicine, energy and agriculture, but also in all areas of political and social life. Subjected to these scientific laws, nothing is ever satisfactory.

Likewise, we're not talking about legitimate trade between men, but about an economy at the service of a globalist financial oligarchy, which pumps out all the wealth and enslaves individuals in a consumer society based on the triumph of individual desire, selfishness and the imposition of the law of the strongest, the smartest, the fattest, to the detriment of the least endowed and the least adapted.

Several things follow from this:

◊ A single, rationalist, materialistic, externalized and superficial way of thinking, universally widespread and progressively imposed on all cultures, traditions and ways of thinking. In the long term, this will ensure the disappearance of all humanity's ancient traditions, of all deep, transcendent and subtle culture, of all humanity's noble dreams. Philosophy and psychology will be entirely rationalized, and all depth and transcendence will be removed. The best of art and poetry will disappear. Spirituality will be forced underground. Human beings will be standardized, assimilated to thinking machines particularly suited to their enslavement and exploitation.

◊ The legitimization and generalization of individual and collective selfishness. This will encourage division, aggression and violence. And in response, a greater need for security, with the gradual abolition of individual freedom.

◊ The disappearance of any depth, of any meaning, apart from personal interest, the disappearance of any order, organization, harmony, knowledge or technique at the service of individual and collective well-being. For official technological progress is today carefully endorsed, selected and limited by the System, replacing genuine progress in the physical and psychic well-being of mankind. And this leads to the elimination of any higher or deeper research, any intuitive or feminine, selfless action, any authentic philosophy or spirituality that might challenge, contradict or threaten it.

That's why the more this model of thinking and lifestyle spreads, the greater the need to meditate will become in that part of the population that has cultivated its consciousness enough to no longer be fooled, hypnotized by the mirages of power and spurious technologies. For the true human being cannot fulfill his or her life without giving it deep meaning. For these people, centering, internalization and meditation are a necessity, similar to the pilgrim's thirst in the desert.[1]

The most widespread objective of meditation is the search for connection with a higher, spiritual, universal, transcendent reality, dimension or presence. It responds to a need, not a duty. It is usually expressed through prayer, oraison, invocation, contemplation, devotion, adoration, the cultivation of silence, meditation, but also the search for a relationship with nature, with what is vast, the beautiful, the good, joy, love, selfless action or knowledge.

Transcendence is built through *elevation* and *depth*. By creating a relationship with the spiritual dimension of the individual and cosmic "I" above and the Psychic Being in the depth of the heart, it balances the expansion of the ego, corollary to the expansion of prâna and consciousness. Without transcendence and transformation, neither expansion nor enjoyment can guarantee the right development of the individual and spiritual life.

Increase your resources

Our world has changed. True, but we still face the same difficulties and dangers that confronted human beings in the Middle Ages, such as epidemics[2] or incessant wars[3]. We enjoy a high degree of material security,

---

1. Meditation will become inaccessible to inoculated people, immersed in an artificial world and a powerful electromagnetic fog.

2. We fear we've entered an era of perpetual epidemics!

3. It has to be said that many countries are in a state of war. As for health, the situation will soon be so catastrophic, combined with the hopeless treatments of modern medicine, that we may come to envy the medicine of the root peoples.

food self-sufficiency and even a certain material abundance. Yet we are not living in happiness, inner calm, full vitality and harmonious emotional abundance, and health levels everywhere are steadily deteriorating.

Our vital force, which is great in youth, rapidly diminishes as the years go by, and our energies and interests are inevitably dulled.

Our scientists and experts, with the approval of our elders, will tell us that all this is normal and that everything in the universe follows the sacrosanct law of entropy.[1]

But there is a contradiction in the fact that the energy of the universe or of Nature appears to us to be unlimited. And there are exceptions to this supposedly inescapable entropy. For example, crudivorism considerably raises the level of individual vitality, and the practice of respirianism[2] raises this level to a superhuman scale, since the individual now needs only a few short hours of sleep and enjoys a permanent psychic and energetic abundance, extra-sensory qualities, new physical qualities and a return to total health.

Similarly, through the practice of yoga, energetic or meditative disciplines, the adept also discovers access to exceptional vitality, to heightened states of consciousness, experiences a capacity to constantly push back one's limits and discovers ever higher vibratory levels.

We can see that there are indeed two levels of existence.

The first is linked to a conventional, normal Nature, defined in a usual representation in relation to the satisfaction of basic needs, precisely those that are exacerbated by the manipulative strategies of our elites and all the circles of power that gravitate in the human sphere. *Panem et circenses*[3]. But also circumscribed within the field of consciousness, where dualities are the rule, and where the body's sensory system constitutes the ultimate reference point[4], the ultimate truth, as within the general frame of reference of Science.

---

1. In a rational, anthropocentric representation, entropy is synonymous with disorder and impoverishment. But in a broader, more conscious representation, it expresses a law of exchange, a transformation.

2. Respirianism: when the individual no longer eats and feeds on prâna.

3. The formula of the Romans, who had already understood everything about politics: bread and circuses".

4. Expressed another way: "the ultimate truth is the sensitivity of the body", this shows the aberration of a simian way of thinking that wants to rule the world!

The second level of existence is revealed when the individual is no longer satisfied by basic needs and personal desires and ambitions, and begins to be inhabited by values that are more subtle, more complex, more vast, more universal, more essential. And then he has to make a "quantum leap, he has to be ready to give up his old values and step into the void to move into the other world. It's difficult, it can be agonizing, but if he holds on to his aspiration, it will carry him to the other shore, step by step or suddenly, depending on his nature and the strength of his need.

This other level of existence, consciousness and energy is attuned, connected, harmonized to the Whole, to universal unity, to the Unified Field of Consciousness/Energy, to a representation in which everything is possible, a world, an Aether whose only limits are those we give it and whose law is plenitude, bliss, ecstatic satiety—or again: perfection, unlimited fulfillment.[1]

This other world, which we call "spiritual" and whose term has been so overused, and which arouses so much mistrust, will perhaps have to be renamed to tame modern man, conditioned to be rational, materialistic, atheistic, agnostic, incredulous, skeptical by habit, selfish and intolerant, adapted for conformity, the short term, and driven ever more towards his most basic needs and desires. Let's not forget that even today, inner vision, contact with the invisible world and the mystical quest are considered psychotic delusions punishable by a psychiatric hospital and a chemical straitjacket!

But apart from the search for transcendence, there is another reason to meditate today, and it's directly linked to the toxic environment created by these new technologies and the growing pressure that the System exerts on the people who fatten the financial elites and transnational corporations. This pressure is expressed in increasingly difficult working conditions, a constant reduction in purchasing power, the dehumanization of professional and administrative life, and an increasingly virtual and limited relational and cultural life, accompanied by an incessant bludgeoning of falsified, faked and manipulated information, omnipresent in the media, which floods the human brains of the planet twenty-four

---

1. This is the great challenge of our time and of post-liberalism, with the transition to what we call superunity and Free Energy, which will express itself not only in the energy field, but in all areas of life.

hours a day, whereas fifty years ago, this took the time of a radio bulletin or reading the newspaper.

In addition to this mental and psychic stress, which constantly rises and systematically occupies our consciousness, drastically limiting our time for reflection, our free time and proportionally amputating all our freedoms, there is a powerful vibratory stress that is growing exponentially.

Electromagnetic, energetic and psychic pollution1

Electromagnetic, electronic and computer technology – and soon Artificial Intelligence (AI) – has developed extremely rapidly. Like all technologies, it was supposed to free human beings from their most thankless, repetitive and tedious tasks, and usher in a new era of leisure and culture. Today, we can see that we have been brilliantly deceived, that it leads to unemployment, loss of human dignity, exploitation and enslavement, already perfectly described fifty years ago in *Brave New World* or in the *Big Brother* concept. Not only has it been used for purposes that could be described as diabolical, but, like all technologies born of this way of thinking about the exploitation of Nature and mankind, it has been manufactured in an artificial, chaotic mode of production, in opposition to the harmonious laws of Nature, and it is only logical that it should produce harmful influences and adverse consequences. The same applies to the synthetic chemicals used in medicine, all of which generate toxic side-effects. There is a breakdown in harmony between artificial products and Nature – in this case, the human body.

And yet, this was not inevitable. We've often observed that the same devices built by different manufacturers don't emit the same degree of electromagnetic pollution, and some don't emit any at all.

We have the technology to match our consciousness

Electromagnetic or electronic technology, or even chemistry that incorporates a harmonious vision of Nature, would emit no pollution, and their influence or radiation could even be beneficial to living organisms. We develop science and technology that are connected to our mental

1. Not taking electromagnetic pollution into account when practicing a discipline linked to a subtle, energetic dimension of the human being, such as yoga, shows a lack of awareness and sensitivity, and reveals a major absence of coherence.

representations. We don't know it, but it makes perfect sense. It's simply a fuller, more complete logic. It's not rationality itself that's at issue, but the limits within which we enclose this logic; it's the depth, breadth and elevation, in a word the quality and subtlety of our vision and intention that matter for the construction of our world and ourselves.

In addition to the high-voltage lines that criss-cross our countryside, we now have hundreds of thousands of relay antennas to power our computers, mobiles, peripherals and all our connected objects with increasingly powerful frequencies. We've now reached 5G – which will considerably increase the number of antennas. And smart meters, known as *Linky* in France, will undoubtedly, along with increased technological connectivity, bring us all more pollution and virtual life, but above all will be an indispensable link in the global system of surveillance and control that Edward Snowden has denounced. Financial elites, the military-industrial complex, pharmaceutical companies and multinationals, to which we can now add GAFAM[1] have infiltrated political spheres and are imposing their pernicious laws on states and citizens.

An electromagnetic haze that is becoming ever denser, especially in cities, and increasingly harmful to body and mind, is spreading everywhere and getting bigger. And we ourselves are installing a Trojan horse for this technology that is destroying us, with our cell phones, computers and peripherals, set-top boxes, TV decoders – and our Wi-Fi and Bluetooth to spread radiation to every room in our house, the room where we sleep or our children's bedroom.

Electromagnetic pollution creates a vibratory chaos that disrupts the harmony of the body's functions, leads to permanent stress, chronic fatigue, insomnia, headaches, attacks all the weak points of our health and undermines our endocrine system day after day, until all the individual's defenses collapse, forbidding the slightest contact with electromagnetism. This is electro-hypersensitivity.

Let's not forget that all our cells, as well as all our water molecules (which account for of our bodies!) and our DNA, function solely through electromagnetism. Without electromagnetism, there's no chemistry, no production of proteins[2], hormones or red blood cells, and nothing can func-

---

1. Google, Apple, Facebook, Amazon, Microsoft, the giants of the Web.
2. There are 8 billion chemical operations per second in the human body!

tion straight in the body's mechanics. And it's this very basis of the body's functioning that is under attack and disrupted, twenty-four hours a day.

But there's more to body pollution than meets the eye, because electromagnetic pollution also has a deleterious influence on our vitality and psyche. And we don't usually talk about this. Homeopaths, on the other hand, are aware of the hierarchy of symptoms, and have given priority to mental and psychological symptoms because they know that they have the greatest impact on the overall health of the human being, and that if left to run their course, illness will inevitably spread to the physical body.

What happens when mental and psychic energies are systematically disrupted and weakened? It's the very engine of the system that's affected, because the brain manages all our functions, the mind is the individual's guide and vitality is its energy. As a result, stress spreads, intellectual fatigue sets in, confusion appears, discernment fades, the mental machine slows down and goes haywire, further disrupted by physical pain in the head and eyes, and depression sets in. The resulting professional, relational and domestic problems make the situation even worse.

So they tell us, the scientific experts in the pay of the multinationals, champions of bad faith and manipulation, that there are no problems, that electromagnetic pollution doesn't exist, with laboratory experiments to back them up, or that they respect the standards of governmental organizations – which they themselves have imposed and whose thresholds they are constantly pushing back. We know their lies and the perversity of their arguments and their communication and development strategies, which they have been expressing for fifty years in every environmental, food and health scandal.

And here, let us emphasize that Science recognizes neither Life nor Consciousness, and that its protocols have been developed to study, *in laboratories*, the laws of matter, a matter that they have enclosed in a dogmatic representation to which it must obey.

Science denies the existence of universal energy. It gets away with it by showing a colossal reservoir of energy at the origin of creation, during a Big Bang that nothing explains. But the universe would have been extinct long ago if the creation of energy had not been accompanied by the preservation of energy. Brahma, the Creator, Vishnu, the Preserver and Shiva, the Destroyer. These are the three indispensable movements of energy in the universe.

How then can Science understand anything about a living, conscious being, when emotion is produced by a gland and thought by a neuron? If Science were right, how can we explain the fact that it has been unable for – let's say two centuries – with all the gigantic human and financial resources at its disposal, to understand and cure diseases, even a simple flu? And why is it that the more science and technology develop, the deeper human beings sink into psychological misery[1] and permanent stress? I smell a rat. There's something to be understood, but we know that there's none so deaf as he who won't hear! So let's not be impressed by their rhetoric and the arrogance of those who position themselves as the holders of knowledge.

And let's not be afraid of reviving the wisdom of ancient traditions, which were based on the experience of multiple generations who didn't have synchrotrons, but at least a sincerity and common sense that our decision-makers can no longer be credited with. Perhaps one day we'll realize that we don't need a synchrotron or a gas crystallograph to understand the workings of Nature, microscopic or macroscopic, because consciousness can know and become everything. But we're not there yet, and why not also use a telescope or electron microscope (preferably of the Raymond Rife type) if that will help us, while we await the miracle of the development of a science of consciousness. All kinds of technologies exist, some of them more subtle and more compatible with expanded consciousness, and it's only natural that they should develop as part of the evolution of matter.

We're all familiar with the allegory of the frog in a cauldron of hot water who doesn't realize he's cooking, because the temperature of the water rises very slowly, then his attention softens with the hotter water and finally he can't escape because he's already half-cooked. This is the methodology of electromagnetic pollution. It's also the ideal strategy for enslaving a people.

Is it too late? Rationally speaking, if we place ourselves in the usual field of coherence, the answer is yes, without a doubt. But if we place

---

1. Or, more precisely, the misery of conscience.

ourselves in the other representation, that of the unity and soul of the world, of the universal quantum field, then everything is always possible at any moment, whatever the catastrophic situation. But we know that the greater the difficulty, the more resources we'll have to accumulate, and the greater our motivation and commitment.

> *What will we feed our souls on," exclaimed a yogi[1] from India, speaking of this technological and societal evolution?*

That's why we have to position ourselves and place ourselves deliberately and totally on the light side if that's what we want. That's why meditation becomes even more essential. But beware! If our bodies are put to the test, in a context that's hard to avoid, we'll tend to escape even further with our consciousness, into the heights, surrendering to life and the world.

On the other hand, if we don't want to abandon our bodies, our life energies and our dreams of accomplishment in the face of adversity, we'll have to make Nature our ally and reveal her deepest powers within and around us, for her resources are powerful and radiate legitimately. Yes, it is legitimate to resist oppression and to exist in the deepest law of our being.

This is why we must not turn our backs on the life force, and why breathing techniques will help us to unite the energies of our nature and the expansion of our consciousness. That's why we must increase all our resources, those belonging to Nature, but also those in the spiritual realm, for they are the most powerful. And we will cultivate the vibratory approach of breathing for the growth of consciousness as much as for the expansion of our vitality.

Mastering thought and image

To paraphrase a quote by Sri Aurobindo,

> *Meditation methods exist to bring us to the threshold where an angel will take us by the hand to take us beyond the horizon.*

---

1. Swami Chidvilâsananda, called Gurumayi by his disciples.

Among these methods, whether for raising our consciousness or for gathering resources, mental silence is unquestionably one of the most powerful, because it opens the door to all the powers of the Supraconscious.

But before we can enter this powerful silence[1], we need to master **the state of non-thought** (and absence of image) and the position of witness, of neutral observer, of non-reaction.

Human beings think through images or thoughts. It depends on our nature. It's the lot of all mankind. And this may come as a surprise, because in collective representation, the mind thinks only by thought. The image may seem to belong to a more rudimentary mind, but appearance is deceptive, because the image is more powerful than thought. Besides, don't the Orientals say, *"A picture is worth a thousand words"*?

In fact, the image – which the academic way of knowing ignores and perhaps even despises – is indispensable for exploring inner worlds and expressing the complexity and wealth of information of the Higher Mind.

The sticky invasion of images and thoughts occupies all the space in our consciousness, and unrolls the litany of the incessant fluctuations of ordinary life. By stopping this uninterrupted flow of thoughts and images, once the surprise and fear of the unknown have passed, the processes of the Deep Mind and Supraconscious begin, heralding the sensory and conceptual revolution of a consciousness that discovers the illusion of its limits.

What's more, mental silence brings an accelerated development of consciousness (seen from the classical meditation side), but also of consciousness-strength (seen from the dynamic meditation side), and we know that Consciousness and Prâna are among the greatest individual human resources we can all access.

Mental silence truly represents the adventure of a limitless evolutionary vision and the wisdom of humanity's dreams. It is the radical means of access to a luminous superhumanity, which can serve the adept of transcendence as much as the builder of a new man and a new world. For, as we have emphasized, silence has two faces, like Janus: static silence,

---

1. It is powerful, but even more so if we connect it to life, for it then becomes a Consciousness-Force.

which quickly slips away beyond the world[1], and dynamic silence, which gives access to the higher levels of the mind and the universal, giving us the means to transform life.

In the next volume, we'll take a closer look at some of these methods. Here, we'll see that breathing will help us get started and give us many opportunities to cultivate the state of non-thinking.

Integral yoga

First of all, it should be noted that the term "*integral*" does not mean that it uses all the techniques belonging to the different forms of yoga, or even that it can be defined solely by the integration of the yogas of Knowledge, Devotion and Works.

Integral Yoga, which Sri Aurobindo explored and described, certainly includes the objectives of these three expressions of spirituality, but it also fully includes the two passive and dynamic representations of the Divine, Consciousness and Energy, Shiva and Shakti, which express themselves in the ideal of the liberation of individual consciousness, but also in the transformation of the human being and the World.

For we note that today, with few exceptions, Tantra and Vedanta aim and speak only of liberation, and very few systematically go through all the rungs of the hierarchy of consciousness, which remains the only way to unite high and low.

> "*Oh, Seers of Truth... Make your way to That which is Immortal; knowers of secret plans, form the steps by which the gods attained immortality.*" —Rig Veda

Likewise, in general, mystics in all traditions focus exclusively on the Divine within, the little eternal flame which, although it often expresses itself in the world, does not recognize itself in the world and has no desire

---

1. The silence of the inner self can also draw us irresistibly into the heart of the unfathomable mystery of existence and bliss. Once you've had a taste of it, it's hard to conceive of any other spiritual goal. The balance between a static and a dynamic spirituality is complicated. The simplest solution is to favor the dynamic form until such time as it seems indispensable. Let's also add that this double silence can come, as we know, from the top of the head, but also from the deep Heart.

to transform it.[1]

Boddhisatvas return to help their spiritual brothers, but they never return to change the laws of suffering and ignorance. They don't come back to heal or transform the roots of the Earth's problem, responsible for the fact that all those who develop their consciousness decide to leave it, to flee it, and finally to betray it.

Sri Aurobindo's answer to the problem that forever divides inner and outer life, Soul and world, is twofold.

First of all, we must definitively accept and integrate these two aspects, inner and outer, and no longer oppose them. This can be done by relying on the dynamic part of the individual Divine, which he called "Psychic Being", as we have seen, but also on Shakti, the dynamic aspect of the Divine. Let's not forget that it is the product of the encounter between the eternal Soul and an individual consciousness launched into human history.

The second answer lies in the transcendence of this synergy of the static (Shiva) and dynamic (Shakti) Divine in a new consciousness/energy, which he called "supramental", capable of reinitializing human life in a higher law, with a transformation, not only of the conditions of life on Earth dependent, no longer on the law of dualities and oppositions, but of unity, but also of the transformation of matter itself liberated from Unconsciousness and Ignorance, an illuminated matter as it were.

From these summits of the Universal Spirit, a new evolutionary principle is incarnated, a fourth, Supramental principle, after those of Matter, Life and Mind.

---

1. We are referring here to the 2 houses of the Soul, the individual Divine in the Heart: (1) the eternal flame, static, non-evolving, the support of static spirituality and (2) the Psychic Being, the evolving, dynamic form, whose purpose is the realization of divine consciousness in the individual and the expression of this perfection in human nature and the world.

II
A NEW MEANING
TO EARTHLY LIFE

The Psychic Being[1] and its realization

Here, we need to make a few clarifications about Sri Aurobindo's spiritual representation, and in particular about the spiritual consciousness in the Human being, which the Indian tradition calls the Conscious Being, the Purusha.

What could be more human than man?

Humanism has a greater universality and incarnation than religious charity and compassion, or the hidden ideals of socialism or even economic liberalism. Humanist philosophy is at the heart of the human being. But it is the Psychic Being who is at the heart of humanism, and it is he who is its meaning and hidden cause.

> "*The Divine is all the knowledge we must acquire, all the power we must obtain, all the love we must become, all the perfection we must achieve, all the harmonious and progressive balance we must manifest in light and joy and all the new and unknown splendors we must realize.*" —The Mother

---

1. From the Greek psyché, soul.

The Soul and the Psychic Being

The concept of the soul in religious tradition is imprecise. In Indian tradition, and in particular as interpreted by Sri Aurobindo, the soul can mean either the eternal, unchanging divine spark formed by the cosmic Self, the seed that gives birth to the Psychic Being, or the Psychic Being itself. Moreover, the soul represents the individual form of the Divine, which also possesses a universal and transcendent form. While it is conceivable that the universal Divine (*Âtman*) inhabits a body, which is precisely the universe, it is also possible to say that the individual Divine (*Jivâtman*) creates an emanation, a spiritual personality, the Psychic Being, which incarnates in a human body over the course of multiple lives.

The formation of individual souls or divine entities has a purpose. Souls were not created for Heaven, but for Earth, not for the universal, but for the individual.

The two stages of soul formation

In the beginning, the individual Divine creates a seed (an emanation), which is the divine spark. It is eternal, perfect and therefore non-evolving. When this seed of light is immersed in terrestrial manifestation, it interacts with Nature and forms around itself a consciousness, then a divine conscious being in the making, which Sri Aurobindo calls the Psychic Being.

There are two stages in this training process.

The first step is the creation of this divine individuality or Psychic Being. In the mineral, vegetable and animal kingdoms, it is more a question of an **influence** that can **be** all the more organized the more evolved the body it inhabits, but in the human being, a true being, an individual consciousness, takes birth, structures itself and culminates after many rebirths in a fully formed, organized being, unique in its differences from other Psychic Beings, conscious of itself and of its divine filiation, entirely master of the human consciousness and nature that is its envelope and becomes its instrument.

Indeed, once fully formed—which takes, perhaps, countless lifetimes—the Psychic Being comes to the forefront of human nature and takes control of the individual. And it can be said that many exceptional human beings, remarkable for their character and actions, women and men, are exceptional because they are on the threshold of this individual human revolution, Psychic Liberation[1]. And this is the only coherent explanation.

The second phase of training, once the Psychic Being has taken control of his instrument, is not limited. It can continue indefinitely. But it is concomitant with its expression in the terrestrial world. It is therefore in this second phase that its true purpose is revealed: **the expression of the Divine in terrestrial nature,** and consequently **its transformation, with** each soul or Psychic Being expressing a certain divine perfection, and the multiplicity of souls each enriching and completing this multiplicity of expression and action in their own way.

Within this divine expression on Earth, we can still distinguish two modes: the first is the expression of the Purusha or static divine principle of consciousness, and the second is the expression of energy and power, of the dynamic divine principle. Not all souls are destined to engage in action as such, but all radiate and are called upon to express the different facets of the Divine.

The two principles of Psychic Being
Individuality and unity

We can distinguish two principles present in the development of the Psychic Being: uniqueness and unity. All souls are one in their essence and unique in their expression. On the one hand, we have the principle of individuation and individuality, linked to the qualities of existence and consciousness in the individual and developing uniqueness in the expression of his consciousness and in his nature.

On the other hand, we find the principle of unity, since the soul stems directly from universal unity: individual consciousness leaves behind its egocentric, selfish orientation, opening up to the diversity and unity of beings and things in a growing intimacy, an identification through deep, spiritual recognition, leading to the perception of unity and the expression of love.

1. Psychic liberation is a true spiritual experience and realization, even if we may consider, in a rational approach, that the realization of universal consciousness is more important than the realization of the individual Divine.

In this concept of soul, we understand that it has two facets: the seed, the heart, the center, **the spark**, eternally in unity – from which emerges its expression, this dynamic, evolving and unique divine being: **the Psychic Being**.

The two traps

In the yoga of the realization of the Psychic Being, there are many obstacles, but they are generally linked to two parts of human nature: the ego and the desire-soul.

The desire-soul, so called by Sri Aurobindo, which is not the true soul, but a kind of personality created by the life force within us and which replaces the true riches of the soul. We could describe it as the essence and collection of the multiple desires of our nature.

The ego, which is the appearance of individuality, *a representation*, a self-image, an artificial and superficial construction. Representation, it should be emphasized, is neither a sensation nor, even less, an experience of the self.

The ego is the shadow and projection in human nature of spiritual individuality; it corresponds to a limited image of ourselves, formed by our personal experience and conditioning, on the mental, vital or physical plane, and with which we identify ourselves. The ego therefore assumes a triple form: mental, vital and physical.

We receive information, we sort it, we formulate it, we sort it again, we analyze it and relate it to others, we organize it and finally we react or act. On the mental plane, we receive information in the form of representations; on the vital plane, we receive it through our vital and emotional sensitivity, through our impressions, and we express reactions to this information; on the physical plane, we receive it through our sensations. In this way, the ego expresses itself in the form of representations, emotions, perceptions, impressions, sensations and reactions.

The ego thus becomes a real entity, a living creation of our own mind, influencing our representations and sensibility as much as our behavior and actions. We will react favorably if the image of ourselves reflected back to us is pleasant or flattering; we will react unfavorably if it is threatened, diminished or perverted in our eyes.

But above all, the ego takes the place of our true identity, our original individuality, our true self.

Sri Aurobindo invites us not to seek to destroy or eliminate the ego, but to transform, broaden, deepen and elevate it. By enlarging, elevating and deepening it, the self-image gradually gives way to the true self, the origin and essence of the principle of individuality.

> *The ego is a particular and necessarily partial representation of oneself, at once conceptual, psychically sensitive and sensory, expressing itself in a receptive and reactive sensibility. But the great characteristic of the ego is the processing of all this information from a (single) point of reference, which is oneself.*

The dynamic vital and the soul-of-desire

The sensory vital, the dynamic vital and the emotional vital[1] are the 3 orientations of the life force within us.

Of these three orientations, the most central is the vital dynamic. This is where the main seat of life energy, Prâna, is located, at the Manipûra chakra in the belly. This is where we distinguish the two divisions of prâna: *physical prâna*, attached to the life and functioning of the physical body, and *psychic prâna*, which gives impetus and energy to our emotional and mental being, either in their own sphere of activity, or for action through the body. Physical prâna is linked to the Mûlâdhâra and Swâddhisthâna chakras, while psychic prâna is linked to the Manipûra and Anâhata chakras. But, like everything else in the field of great Nature, there are relationships in every sense.

The proper action of psychic prâna," explains Sri Aurobindo, "is pure possession and enjoyment. Enjoyment of thought, will, action, dynamic impulse, the result of action, feelings, sensations, and also enjoyment through them of objects, people, life and the world.

This quest is realized through desire, through what Sri Aurobindo called "the soul of desire".

"The root of desire is the vital lust that seeks to seize what we believe we don't have. It's life's limited instinct to possess and satisfy. It creates

---

1. They correspond to the three chakras: Swâddhisthâna, Manipûra and Anâhata.

a sense of lack: first the simple lust of hunger, thirst and lust, then the hungers, thirsts and psychic lusts of the mind. And desire introduces the whole game of attraction and repulsion.

"Psychic prâna invades the sensory mind and introduces the unquenchable thirst for sensations; it invades the dynamic mind with the lust for authority, possession, domination, success and the satisfaction of all impulses; it fills the emotional mind with the desire to satisfy sympathies and antipathies, to satiate love and hatred ; it brings the retreats and panics of fear, the tensions and disappointments of hope, imposes the tortures of pain, the sudden fevers and brief excitements of joy; it makes intelligence and the intelligent will accomplices in all this chaos and transforms... the will into a will to lust, and intelligence into a greedy, biased, groping pursuer of limited, hasty opinions and militant prejudices.

Desire is the root of all sorrow, all disappointment, all affliction, for although it has the feverish joy of pursuit and satisfaction, it constantly brings tension into being and introduces toil into its pursuit and gain, hunger, conflict, rapid subjection to fatigue, a feeling of limitation, dissatisfaction, rapid disappointment with all one's acquisitions, unhealthy and unremitting stimulation, turmoil, anxiety.

> *We must therefore distinguish between will and desire, discern between the inner will to bliss and the lust and lust of the body and mind. Otherwise, we are condemned to either kill the life force, give license to the gross will to live, or compromise between the two. —Synthesis of yogas*

In the course of evolution, the life force impulse will diversify and adopt ever more varied forms of expression, eventually covering the whole range of our impulses and desires, interests, emotions and actions. It's natural for the life force to expand and conquer all areas of existence. In fact, it's the first principle of this vital being to grow, amplify, prosper and conquer.

The natural impulse of the vital dynamic is therefore energy, movement; it loves action, change, diversity of objects, situations and encounters. It is under the influence of *Rajas*[1], the kinetic principle. He loves intensity

1. The three principles of Nature in Indian tradition are : *Tamas*, inertia, *Rajas*, kinetic energy and *Sattwa*, superior balance.

and extremes; he's not concerned with good or truth. Its characteristics are: growth, the quest for possession and power, enjoyment, conquest, domination and mastery.

The vital being is therefore the place of all mixtures, but also, let's not forget, the means of fulfillment and realization in life. It's in the first years of life that we can best observe the power of the uncontrolled vital force in children. It's in adolescence and early adulthood that we can best appreciate this dynamism, this taste for enterprise, conquest and mastery, fulfillment and growth or inner and outer evolution.

By living in the world, we cannot afford to eliminate this delicate power to live and handle. And if we are not satisfied in this vital and emotional realm, in a vague compromise that solves nothing and consigns the human being to a mediocre life, with no real elevation or depth, all that remains is for us to get to know ourselves and grasp our nature as intelligently as possible. These means and methods exist, in a coherence that doesn't stifle life, but on the contrary fulfills it by transforming it.

Perfecting psychic prâna

Here Sri Aurobindo describes the future perfection of this life impulse in the human being:

"The soul of desire must accept all impulses and orders, whatever they may be, which come to it from Spirit through the channel of a still mind and a pure heart. Finally, it must also accept the result of the impulse, whatever it may be: the greater or lesser enjoyment, full or nil, dispensed to it by the Master of our being.

"*Nevertheless, possession and enjoyment are its law, its function, its utility, its swadharma[1]. The soul-of-desire is not meant to be destroyed, nor mortified, nor numbed in its receptive power, nor dull, nor repressed, mutilated, inert or void.*

"The first necessity is the perfecting of vital capacity in the mind... Most of the qualities we need for our perfection – courage, realizing will power in life (strength of character, force of personality) depend to a great extent on abundant psychic prâna to have full spring and vigor in their dynamic action.

---

1. Swadharma is the right law of a being, an energy, an element of Nature.

"But along with this abundance must come joy, clarity and purity in the psychic vital being. This dynamism must not be a restless or excited force, stormy, capricious or brutally passionate.

"Finally, the third condition for the perfection of psychic prâna: it must take its position in complete equality.

The desiring soul must be rid of its clamors, its insistence or the inequality of its desires so that these can be satisfied in a fair and balanced way and in the right manner, and finally it must purge them completely of their desire character and change them into impulses of the divine Ananda[1].

"*It must have a full power of possession, a joyous power of enjoyment, a triumphant power of pure, divine passion and enthusiasm.*

"*Fullness, purity and clear joy, equality, the ability to possess and enjoy, such is the fourfold perfection of psychic prâna.*" – *The Synthesis of the Yogas*

The functions of the Psychic Being

The Psychic Being thus assumes different functions.

◊ He is *the awakener* and works on every plane to help everyone awaken to Consciousness and Truth.

◊ He is *the Binder*: he is there to create the relationship between the Divine and the human being, between universal Intelligence and everyday life.

◊ As such, it is *the "evolver"*: it introduces the infinite into the finite, generating evolution, progress and perfection. The soul's role is also to make man a true being.

◊ He is therefore also *the Guide* who organizes life.

◊ Finally, it is *the Center of* Ego Unification.

The powers and qualities of the Psychic Being

◊ The power of progress

The Psychic Being is psychological firmness, the opposite of sluggishness, slackness, laziness, abandonment of effort, submission to fate, discouragement and depression. It expresses strength, mastery and sovereignty, struggle and victory over the forces of darkness, unconsciousness and ignorance. It brings us the energy of progress, evolution, growth, be-

---

1. Ânanda, bliss.

coming, personal development, continual education, unlimited growth of consciousness and the ceaseless perfecting of nature.

"If one succeeds in consciously uniting with one's Psychic Being, then one can always be in that state of receptivity, inner joy, energy, progress..." – The Mother, *Interviews*

◊ Knowledge of the heart. This is the "little voice", the infallible discerner of truth.

◊ Peace and serenity.

◊ Contentment and equality of soul, non-desire at the heart of the world.

◊ Sweetness, fullness, joy.

◊ Gratitude and compassion.

"Compassion and gratitude are essentially psychic virtues. They appear in consciousness only with the participation of the Psychic Being in active life" – The Mother

◊ Unity and love

The realization of one's Psychic Being
The three stages
The first step is to find your Psychic Being. For some people, the influence is alive, and all you have to do is let it grow or learn to concentrate in the Heart to contact it at will. The second step is to live with it, in it, to establish an increasingly intimate and strong relationship; the third, to bring it to the forefront of our being, in place of the ego and the mind.

Ideally, there are three other possibilities:

1. To maintain contact with the Psychic Being throughout youth and adolescence, and to build one's life and develop one's individuality under its influence. In view of humanity's current consciousness, we would say that this path belongs to the future.[1]

2. To find someone who has already traveled the road to help us get through these three stages.

3. To cultivate transcendence, centeredness, sincerity, self-awareness, and to consciously participate in building individuality and transforming the ego.

The various philosophical and psychological aspects of the Yoga of the

1. It is totally dependent on the degree of evolution of individual consciousness and Karma.

Psychic Being were developed by Sri Aurobindo and The Mother and included in their written works.

It's mainly the technical aspect that we present and develop in this book. The realization of the Psychic Being is the first step in his yoga.[1]

The transformation of consciousness and nature

The Yoga of the Psychic Being includes two parallel paths of evolution: that of consciousness and that of nature.

Experiments are a good thing, but the trouble is that they don't seem to transform nature, they only enrich consciousness.

Harmonizing nature with the inner realization of consciousness, so as not to be divided. – Letters

Transformation in life

How do we move from ego consciousness to Psychic Being? There's a link between the two: the growth and evolution of individual consciousness and individuality. The construction and adventure of individuality.

How do we move from our superficial nature around the ego to that of the Psychic Being? There's a transition between the two, and that's to cultivate the deep nature: deep mental, deep vital, and for people very close to body awareness: the deep physical.[2]

We must also cultivate the influence and presence of the Psychic Being.

We can distinguish four factors that favor the influence and presence of the Psychic Being:

1 – Be receptive to the influence of the Psychic

If we're barricaded inside our ego, closed in our rationalist and materialistic mind, jaded about everything, chasing our desires and locked in our conditioning and habits, how can we be receptive to anything else and in particular to the influence of the Psychic Being? Didn't Christ say: "Become like little children"? And in this sense, for receptivity and open-

1. There are exceptions for individuals whose spiritual destiny is to realize other forms of the Divine without passing through this stage.

2. The deep luminous part of the three bodies has been called by Sri Aurobindo "the subliminal nature". They are the expression of the Psychic Being with the three purushas, mental, vital and physical, symbolized in Tantric symbolism by the three shiva lingams at Mûlâdhâra, Ânahata and Âjnâ chakras.

ness, they are our models.

It should be noted, however, that receptivity to the Psychic Being is a passive attitude; we can also cultivate a conscious and voluntary attitude to connect with it, as, for example, in centering.

2 – Calming the surface

Let's emphasize here that, given the conditions in which we live, stress invades every compartment of our nature. The first consequence of our meditations will be to manage it, then heal it.

Sri Aurobindo points out that it's only when the mind and the vital have calmed down that the Psychic Being can exert his influence. Calming the mind and the vital does not mean an episodic movement, but the definitive transformation of the "terrain" of our nature, of its substance, *the citta*. This means moving beyond the human, beyond our desires and passions, our fears and attachments, our emotions and feelings, which are also the result of all the experiences of our past lives[1], going beyond, at least to some extent, our representations and conditioning. This means unmasking the ego and combating selfishness. We need to assimilate our nature and our present life before we can discover what connects all our lives.

This is the path of maturity, of growing inner awareness and strength.

3 – Developing individuality

Individuation is fundamental to psychic fulfillment. When the individual is suggestible and permeable to all environmental influences, without organization or unification around a central consciousness, as we observe in the young child, we are obviously unable to preserve the full presence of the Psychic.

> *True individuality grows around the growth*
> *of consciousness-strength within the individual*

This individuation leads to the unification of the self, and this unification can only take place around the true center, the true personality.

---

1. Which is no mean feat!

Around the ego, there can only be a chaotic assembly of different parts of the superficial nature, forever in conflict with each other. This means unmasking the ego and fighting all forms of egoism.

Individuality leads to maturity: becoming conscious, responsible, the actor of one's own life, autonomous, structured, unified, stable, filled with inner strength.

This means facing up to our nature, facing difficulties and problems, confronting, assimilating, resolving – a permanent school of acceptance and adaptation. In today's world, which encourages all kinds of escape strategies or the search for external or internal tranquility, we need to mobilize strongly to take charge of ourselves and consciously undertake self-transformation. So it's also the opposite of withdrawal, and we might ask ourselves how we can reconcile even moderate internalization or inner silence in this rigid, externalizing world.

But mental silence can exist and grow in the midst of action or in the midst of exchanges and relationships, because, as we've already pointed out, there are two forms of silence: static silence, which is incompatible with action and externalization and is cultivated in classical meditation, and dynamic silence, which is totally compatible with external life and action.

4 – Releasing karma

The fourth condition for the spiritual realization of the Psychic Being is the liberation of karma. It is perhaps the one that conditions the other three.

What does the liberation of Karma mean? It is its assimilation. And what does Karma mean? It seems to be the condensed consequence of all past life experiences. So it goes much further than one might imagine.

Karma liberation, however, cannot be the assimilation of all experiences, all actions, thoughts, emotions, sensations, which, of course, can only be countless. In reality, what we need is the ability to assimilate them, and it seems enough to be able to assimilate just one real trauma from each family. For there are families of experiences, traumas, sensations, fears, reactions, behaviors or actions, mistakes or setbacks.

We've all been victims and victimizers, albeit to varying degrees and sometimes to a greater or lesser extent. Even if we confine ourselves to the main experiences, and most of the time it's the first times we felt and reacted inappropriately that are the most important, because they led to the repetition of the same mistake and the same suffering given or received over sometimes many lifetimes, often even with a crescendo in intensity and magnitude. Likewise, we don't need to relive all the suffering, mistakes or maladaptive or abusive behavior. Only those that have had significant consequences on our own evolution, on others or on the course of human evolution need to be understood and repaired. Many can be dissolved or consumed by divine fire without our having to relive them.

Because the most important thing, we believe, is not to correspond and respond to the laws of a morality, even a cosmic one, but to build maturity within ourselves. And maturity is also the capacity for awareness-strength that enables us to avoid repeating the same mistakes. And consciousness is also the ability to feel and express love, unity and harmony, but also strength and energy, the ability to integrate complex, vast and subtle situations, environments, feelings and concepts. If we've been put on an evolutionary curve, the notion of error must entirely replace the concept of sin. Good and evil, light and shadow, have been and are the tools of our evolution.

Contrary to what some people say, we don't think it's fair to say that we chose our own evolution. We didn't choose our destiny ourselves, and we don't know to what extent we choose the methods and means of traversing this curve of growth of a consciousness-force immersed in space and time! All this is beyond our comprehension and personal power.

This would be the case if we were identified with our soul, and if we were identified with our soul, we'd be at the end of the journey, in its liberation phase.

Responsibility exists, and we must assume the errors and abuses of the aggressor as much as we must free ourselves from the toxic strategies of our victim behavior. We must also grow in inner strength, increase our capacity for enjoyment and mastery, and free ourselves through elevation and balance from the forms of inertia and weakness as much as those of violence.

Evolution also means adhering to the Good. Not the good of our morals (Mother used to say that if we added them all up, we'd be incapable of any action!), but the higher Good that emerges when we move from ego-centric interest to collective interest, and when we move from the short term to a vision that extends far into time and space. For the growth of consciousness is also the recognition and integration of differences, and therefore of the value of the uniqueness of beings and forms. It's also the ability to rise above opposites and dualities, to transcend and harmonize oppositions and contradictions between the individual and the collective. If we are evolving beings, our journey inevitably leads us, albeit more or less slowly, to understand, feel and become a universal being, one with beings, forms and things, one with the Soul of the world.

It's up to the Psychic Being to see and decide when we're ready to choose the path of unity, oneness and universality, so that it can manifest itself fully at the heart of our consciousness, at the center of our nature.

The three methods of resolving karma

We can distinguish three methods for healing karmic problems.

The first is to revisit past situations linked to the trauma we are trying to eliminate, and which originated in our childhood or past lives. This can be achieved through hypnosis, meditation or any other catharsis-inducing method[1]. But resolving the conflict or trauma depends above all on the therapist's ability to awaken in the patient a position of witness, of non-reaction, of transcendence.

The second is to detect in our everyday behaviors, emotions, reactions and tendencies, those that are chronically, i.e. recurrently, maladjusted. And for this, we often need the help of others. And it could even be said that it's in conflict that they're most easily brought to light.

Once they've been made aware, they need to be opposed by a transcendent position of witness, capable of relativizing, understanding, integrating and assimilating. And thus change these behaviours or psychological reactions. This implies a sincere desire to transform oneself, and the ability to integrate the position of witness deeply within oneself.

1. Modern psychotherapies, since the experiments of Stanislav Grof and his colleagues, with psychotropic drugs or holotropic breathing, have invented different methods.

It would seem that using both methods in parallel is the most fruitful.

There's a third, spiritual method, which belongs entirely to the realm of meditation and yoga. This is the elevation of consciousness into the Supraconscious.

For it is a law that whatever goes up must come down.[1]

"The eternal tree has its roots above and extends its branches below," says the Katha Upanishad.

"The future," says Satprem[2], "goes from top to bottom; it descends more and more into our mental fog, our vital confusions, into the subconscious and unconscious night, until it has illuminated everything, revealed everything, cured everything – and finally accomplished everything."

Indeed, every spiritual seeker experiences this alternation of enlightenment and descent[3], which we are often tempted to regard as falls or failures. If we want to push the needle of our compass a little more upwards, or rather, simply, if we want to make the process of transformation more enjoyable, the first thing is to accept the situation and reconsider our view of ourselves. We are more than we think we are, both upwards and downwards. And there's a long road ahead of us, whatever we do. Some may think it's better to take themselves less seriously, and seek to bring a little more lightness into their lives. Others will keep their noses to the grindstone, stubbornly pushing their little cart of misery. When you've been through life, you can always tell yourself that you could have taken a different path!

Nevertheless, we can't help thinking that there must be better strategies for pushing evolution into our daily lives as the years go by without us ever realizing it.

The important thing is to get through, we think, when the going gets tough. Some people today call this congruence. But as we go through difficulties, if the inner fire within us is not extinguished, we notice that an inner strength develops, accompanied by a certain enjoyment in the crossing.

1. Too bad the opposite isn't true!
2. See *Sri Aurobindo or The Adventure of Consciousness*, by Satprem, published by Discovery Publisher.
3. We're always much further down than we are up!

A bit like pushing wheelbarrows day after day[1] develops our muscles and eventually eliminates any unpleasant sensations associated with physical effort. The practice of sport accustoms us to surpassing ourselves, and even when we no longer have the physical capacity, we'll always have the moral strength and passion for physical effort when we know it contributes to our well-being or progress. The same applies to psychic and pranic disciplines, all the more so as they bring their own rewards. We can become accustomed to suffering when we have at our disposal numerous means of overcoming it or of initiating pleasant experiences through the mastery of numerous techniques. It's the idea that not only is there one solution to my problem, but that there are many. This brings about a positive change in our attitude to adversity. And it's always fun to solve a problem when we know we've got something to spare!

That's why we've chosen to multiply the means of personal transformation. But this implies a passion for all these disciplines.

---

1. Or to learn the ropes in music, gymnastics or weightlifting.

III

PREPARATION
FOR MEDITATION

Quickly improve your mental environment

In the early stages of our discipline, we strive to access new states of consciousness, but we've become accustomed to permanent externalization, and the task seems difficult. On the other hand, we're not always in top physical and mental condition – far from it. Some days, we're tired or depressed and can't mobilize ourselves for the practice, or we're in the grip of a stubborn emotion, or we simply can't concentrate. Preparation is not useless.

Through short, accessible exercises, we aim to achieve two objectives. The first is to become capable of modifying the condition of our mind at will. This ability or skill is very useful when we first start practising, but will remain so for many years to come until we have stabilized our inner life. At some point, the exercises will become unnecessary.

The second objective is to prepare for concentration and sitting meditation.

In fact, it's not normal to start practising directly when our mind is in a condition that makes it difficult to centre or internalize. In this case, we need to make a transition, a separation between our outer activities and our sitting. This can be achieved through these exercises, but also through strong motivation, by bringing our aspiration, representation and intention to the surface, or through a small personal ritual if it is sufficiently effective. In fact, we can generally regard these exercises as a ritual to introduce us to the Inner Garden with the right attitude and abilities.

When should you practice?

Meditation can be practised at any time, at home when you're at peace, or when you're in difficulty. But it's when we spontaneously feel like it that the best meditations are guaranteed. Generally speaking, however, the morning is an ideal time, because we can enjoy the benefits all day long, and because morning energies are more dynamic. This is when we realize the need for discipline. Apart from these moments, let's not forget that we can also practice many exercises in bed, between wakefulness and sleep[1]. They will prepare us for sleep, fertilize our insomnia or positively orientate the start of the day.

Finally, in our busy lives, in repetitive or familiar activities, or on public transport, in moments of waiting, we can take advantage of these moments to practice short mental relaxation, balancing or centering exercises.

What should you practice?

We need to start with familiar, easy practice. We each have our "strong points. We need to identify and cultivate them. Recognize the general characteristics of our nature: mental, emotional or at ease in action. We also need to identify the practices that prove effective when we're in difficulty. Let's distinguish between physical, respiratory, energetic, concentration or action-based practices.

For example, a person at ease in the intellectual realm will need to awaken the head chakra, Âjnâ, or its space (Chidâkâsh); an emotional person may find it easy to concentrate in the chest, but on days when they are in an emotional situation, they will need a different approach and different exercises.

We'll see later that it's in everyone's interest to awaken and cultivate the Âjnâ chakra as a priority.

1. This can resolve certain situations in married life or family life.

The liberation of consciousness and the transformation of our nature

We will therefore have two objectives: the liberation of consciousness and the transformation of nature. We'll probably be more tempted to work on consciousness, and it's a basic priority at the beginning to awaken inner awareness, but we mustn't neglect the transformation of our nature.

Consciousness work encompasses everything to do with inner vigilance, including the inner space of the head. Working on our nature corresponds to the transformation of thoughts, images, mental atmospheres, emotions and sensations.

Why so many methods?

This book contains a wide range of exercises. Some are pedagogical tools, tools for looking at ourselves differently, or for taking a first step in an unusual direction and discovering new capacities. Some, perhaps, only need to be practiced once, but with total commitment. But if the exercise is aimed at awakening dormant capacities, certain nâdîs or chakras, and even more so at discovering and establishing inner silence and connection with our deepest Self, it will be necessary to pursue them for weeks, months or years.

> *The multiple approach responds to the diversity of man and life.*

Truth can only be matched by wholeness. Life in all its diversity is the symbol of this wholeness, and it is this diversity that creates the richness of the individual and the universe.

A multiplicity of approaches leads to a multiplicity of experiences. It is necessary to diversify approaches firstly to enable the realization of these two objectives in relation to consciousness and nature, and secondly because the human being himself is multiple and complex, different in nature and personal history, different in difficulties, capacities and objectives. For every human perfection is unique. We often need to change our practice. Changing our method or technique, or changing the way we represent it, while of course maintaining its coherence, reawakens interest and pleasure in our practice. Discipline is slowly killed by habit.

On the other hand, an exclusive method leads to a linear experience that quickly becomes exclusive, i.e. it rejects everything that doesn't fit into its experience. We are quickly tempted to exclude other paths, other methods, other researchers.

> *A multiplicity of approaches leads to a multiplicity of experiences.*

Finally, as we've already pointed out, we can never have too many ways of learning to exist, integrate the world and transform ourselves in an environment where it's very difficult to follow an inner path.

Integrating passive and dynamic methods

The diversity of methods and practices is first and foremost justified by the recognition of the two aspects of reality: one is turned inwards, the other outwards. Attaching importance to only one of these aspects compromises our search for truth, and inevitably leads us down a path that eliminates half of it. Today, humanity is heading for a dead end, with all its attendant suffering and dissatisfaction, forcing us to face up to all the data in the equation of life or disappear. With practice, we'll see that meditation and inner silence can lead us in both directions. By choosing one or the other, the consequences are not the same, and it's by choosing both together that we'll find the solution to fulfilling man both in his inner and outer life.

It's not enough to try and save your soul by entering into inner silence. It's time to understand that the soul is not just a daughter of Heaven. It is married to Heaven and Earth, transfiguring them both. For Heaven can only be fully realized if it is incarnated. The individual Soul has two objectives: the first is to rediscover its full identity by uniting with its divine origin. All spiritualities have stressed this. The second is to progressively express and manifest divine consciousness, fullness, love and perfection. Earth was created to embody the delights of the banquet of the universe, to give substance to the wonders of the Spirit, not to serve as a labyrinth and arena.

This is why we will present methods and practices in the dual light of traditional meditation on the one hand, and dynamic meditation on the other, which establishes the relationship between Heaven and Earth. That said, we must not rank these two approaches. It's a good idea to give priority to dynamic meditation until we've mastered the basics, because we live in the world and generally don't have the stability and balance needed to adhere to an exclusive path of internalization in an entirely outward-looking environment.

However, it's clear that classical meditation, by focusing on consciousness, focuses on the essential, and that this silence of Shiva possesses a powerful magnetism, something that irresistibly attracts us because the closer we get to it, the more we recognize our own home, then feel and realize that it is the Heart of our being.

But it's by mastering both that a new path will emerge, and with it a new power capable of transforming the roots of man and life.

But if we're looking for self-realization in symbiosis with life and the world, in perfecting our nature and respecting the uniqueness of each individual, a multiple approach is necessary.

Is the multiple approach a waste of time?

The multi-faceted approach, with techniques that are both vibratory and psychological, but that also affect different parts of our personality and nature from different angles, will give us the plasticity we need to compensate for and counteract our resistance.

We can liken this to the practice of posture (âsana). If we train exclusively and intensively in back-stretching postures, for example, we'll achieve exceptional back flexibility within a few weeks, but the antagonist muscles will degenerate and we'll see physical and probably also psychological problems appear, as a consequence of a real imbalance. It's the same with any linear technique or execution. On the other hand, if we practice a daily âsana session, taking care to combine all the different families of postures, and balancing stretching and toning, we'll receive all the benefits of our session.

We've often observed this phenomenon with yoga postures, but also by alternating inner techniques, and there it seems that the results are much more profound. And, as with the postures, this doesn't prevent you from insisting more and more each day in one direction. When we take up a particular technique again, after a week or even six months, we always notice progress. This demonstrates that it's possible to practice several techniques alternately, with the advantages of diversity and without the disadvantages of linear practice.

This is because psychological and energetic resistance always lifts after a certain period of practice, and we don't get more results with just one method, however powerful it may be. A technical change allows us to work in a different direction and to advance other parts of our nature, while assimilation continues. Day by day, our receptivity or blockages change.

Of course, in the beginning we need time to master these different techniques, but this disadvantage is more than compensated for by the fact that they are easier and quicker to learn. Indeed, as our inner life and consciousness-strength grow, the effectiveness of the practices increases over time, and experiences or changes in consciousness occur more rapidly. If we become capable of concentrating on one method, the same will soon be true of all the others, and if we master one or two kriyâs well, it will be easy for us to master the others. Eventually, we take pleasure in this diversity and become free to choose according to our mood or need.

However, in all this diversity, certain methods keep coming back. They will prove to be more fundamental, more profound, more in tune with our nature and more effective. A refocusing occurs spontaneously. Diversity doesn't detract from what's essential. Besides, do we need to multiply our techniques unconsciously? A few practices well chosen for their complementarity are sufficient today, and we'll discover others when the time comes.

Finally, the multiple approach is also a help and a safeguard. By comparing different points of view, we can become more aware both of the mechanisms common to different practices and of our own mistakes. By following a single method or an exclusive line of development, we inevitably expose ourselves to all the limitations and deviations associated with it. What's more, as we've seen, the multiple approach prevents us from falling into habit and mechanical repetition. *The instructor will be on his guard against anything that might transform the means into limitations or mechanize practice.* — *The Synthesis of Yogas*

The multi-faceted approach helps us to better understand our own path as well as that of others. It also enables us, when faced with an impasse, to choose a new direction. Sometimes we have to overcome our attachment to our own method of meditation to discover the treasures hidden in others.

What to do on difficult days

On difficult days, we need to remember the areas or exercises in which we excel. What are the practices that make us stronger, whatever the difficulties? They take priority in our practice.

Then we'll proceed with more preparation or steps. We'll choose exercises adapted to our current difficulties to prepare us for inner concentration, or if that's still not possible, we'll choose exercises that restore our balance or improve our state of mind, while leaving more in-depth practice for later. Some days, it might be better to go for a jog first! In any case, a realistic view of our inner condition will be beneficial.

> *From stress to calm and inner peace, from fatigue and inertia to dynamism and mental firmness, from unconsciousness and confusion to clarity and vigilance, from agitation and externalization to stability and internalization, from submission to environment and destiny to autonomy, from withdrawal to openness, receptivity and the adventure of change towards inner freedom, balance, perfection and joy.*

We mark exercises that are essential and particularly effective with three stars (★★★). On the other hand, some of them are difficult. In these cases, it may be useful to first practice the preparatory exercises that are usually described beforehand.

Stars are associated with essential practices.

Practice the most efficient, the essential.

The Practice

IV
IMPROVE
THE INNER CONDITION

Meditation postures

The principles underlying the choice of posture in meditation are rela-
tive. They will necessarily depend on your body's capabilities. But there's
nothing to stop you from training to improve it.

Padmâsana, the Lotus

The best pose—because it's the only one that balances our internal energy perfectly—is Lotus pose, called Padmâsana in India. But it's the most
difficult, especially for us Westerners, with our rigid pelvis and knees.
Remember that the knee joint is the most fragile of all. The half-lotus is
more affordable.

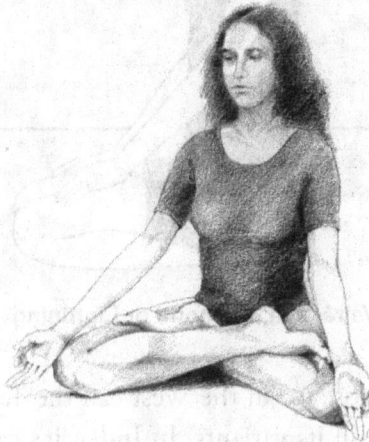

Padmâsana, the Lotus

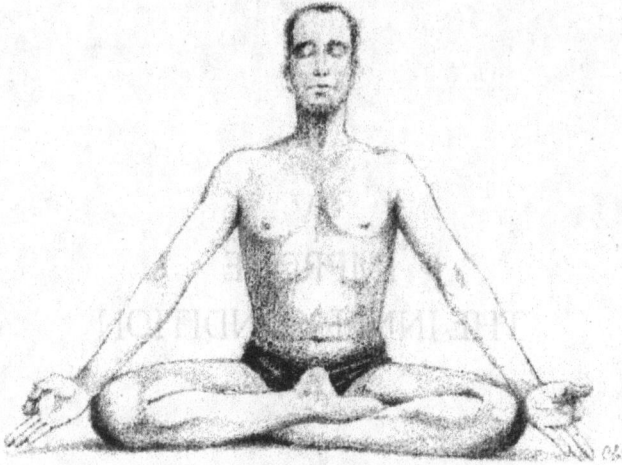

Siddhâsana, the perfect pose

Then comes the Diamond pose, Vajrâsana, adopted for prayer by Muslims and many others of all origins. A cushion or small stool can be placed under the buttocks.

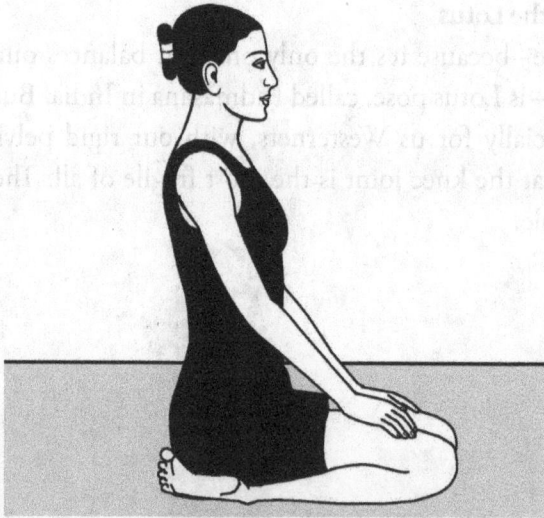

Vajrâsana, Diamond or Lightning

Finally, we find the pose we in the West call the Tailor, the pose of the Egyptian scribe, with all its variants. In India, it's called Sukhâsana, the easy pose. It has a number of disadvantages.

Having said that, what's important is to tilt the pelvis forward, so as to arch the lower back slightly – and this can be achieved with a cushion or possibly a Nordic-style seat -, to clear the chest with the shoulders relaxed and set back, and to keep the head upright and balanced. Sitting on the floor with legs crossed is a better choice, but if the position is too difficult for you, at least at first, sit on a chair with a cushion at the back. Some schools impose a difficult posture, especially for knees[1]. We personally believe that the priority is to work on the mind, and that too much effort of will, leading to stress, is not conducive to meditation, which must combine "masculine qualities, such as vigilance, with "feminine qualities, such as letting go. In any case, train regularly and make your leg joints more flexible, giving priority to the pelvic joints, so that you can later adopt a sitting position on the floor.

A few simple ways

Here are a few simple ways to get rid of stress and regain a positive energetic and psychological state: sport, hot baths, cold or hot foot baths with salt, saunas, massage, singing, neck stretching, postures and, of course, yoga muscle relaxation.

We introduced them in our previous book, *Soothe and Transform Your Mind*.

The eyes and mental relaxation

Today, our eyes are subjected to a double pressure: electromagnetic and light pollution associated with the widespread use of multiple computer screens on the one hand, and the widespread wearing of corrective glasses on the other. In all cases, electromagnetic pollution brings mental and nervous stress, which has repercussions on the eyes. Light from screens also directly assaults the eyes. Wearing glasses, when they are precisely adapted to the wearer's eyesight, relieves eye strain, but prevents accommodation, which inevitably means stronger and stronger glasses. But most of the time, they are designed with a stronger correction to prevent programmed deterioration, and this leads to additional eye strain. Not

---

1. The knees are the weakest link in seated poses.

to mention bifocals or progressive lenses, which seek to replace natural ocular plasticity with artificial correction.

Meditation, and all concentration exercises, also exert mental and ocular tension at the start of practice, and who can say when meditation leads to ocular relaxation? And how can you meditate well when you approach the discipline with stressed, tired eyes and a mind under constant tension?

This is why we believe that eye relaxation has become essential to the practice of meditation, precisely because of the influence of the mind on the eyes and the eyes on the mind.

Among the most important exercises, we recommend :

◊ Firstly, eye relaxation, which means that we need to develop a reflex of awareness of eye tension in active life, and thus generalize eye relaxation.

◊ Mobilization with eyes in every direction

◊ The habit of blinking, especially in front of screens.

◊ Training your eyes to accommodate near ←→ distance. We once knew a 75-year-old woman who still had the perfect vision of her youth. She had practised this last exercise all her life.

It's a discipline that needs to be integrated into life, from youth to old age.

N° 1 – SOFTENING THE EYES

Our eyes are directly linked to our mind. Through the eyes, we can stop our mind by immobilizing the eyes, or soften them to create a break in our intellectual activity and release ocular and mental tension.

In India, it is said that the main cause of deterioration in eyesight is mental tension, which is automatically transmitted to the eye muscles. This has been known since the work of Dr. Bates in 1920, but India has listened, as it has remained close to natural health solutions. In the West, the rationalist approach, coupled with the interests of eyewear manufacturers[1], was bound to be impervious to a natural method of vision correction.

Anyone whose eyesight has deteriorated can regain a few tenths through appropriate eye gymnastics, but this can only bear fruit if eye relaxation

1. For those who doubt it, the most widespread and stable commercial outlets in our towns and cities are pharmacies, **opticians**, insurance companies and bakeries.

accompanies the exercises.

That's why we recommend performing eye movements while exhaling, or remaining aware of what you see in front of you during the movement. Concentrate on what you see uninterruptedly, rather than on the eye movement.

Learn to relax your eyes and correct yourself regularly during the exercises, as well as during the day.

Hold your arm out in front of you and look at your thumbnail. Then move your arm slowly from right to left, up and down, and finally make a semicircle to the right with your right arm and a semicircle to the left with your left arm. As you follow the nail, your eyes move in all directions. Take care not to move your head. Finally, place your thumb on the tip of your nose, then on the middle of your forehead, bringing your gaze up and down. Then relax your eyes.

VARIANT: THE LEMNISCATE ∞★★★

Close your eyes and follow in your imagination the path of a lemniscate (a horizontal figure eight) whose center (the point of intersection) is located between the eyebrows, in the indentation between the nose and the forehead. This point is called *Trikutî*. The trajectory follows the circumference of each eye. Follow the curve as closely as possible for a few moments, then relax your eyes.

Once you've mastered the movement, widen the curve laterally, on the sides, to amplify the relaxation.

N° 2 – EYE RELAXATION

As we've seen, mental tensions embed themselves in the eye muscles, making them rigid and ultimately damaging our vision. This can be compared to the muscular contractions in the back, which exert asymmetrical and prolonged pressure on our vertebrae, distorting our statics and maintaining our cervical, dorsal and lumbar pain. Conversely, any relaxation of the eyes tends to restore the mind to a state of calm and balance.

To relax the eyes, there's just one movement to learn. It's a simple one. When we're tense and uptight, the eyeballs tend to pop forward out of their sockets. In fact, this movement is often caricatured in the surprised expression of certain American cartoon heroes. So, if we want to relax the eyes, we need to perform the opposite movement, bringing the eyeballs back into their sockets.

Lie down, preferably, or sit in an armchair, with your head leaning back. Then let the eyeballs sink into their sockets, concentrating on the weight of the eyes, in a movement of relaxation and dilation. Relaxation then spreads instantly to the back of the neck and the mind.

In the beginning, alternate movements of voluntary tensing and relaxation of the eyes, so as to remember the sensation that you will be able to detect later in your various activities.

N° 3 – WIDEN YOUR EYES

Eye relaxation can be further enhanced by a lateral, outward movement. This is what we see in this exercise.

Here we find the same breath support for our concentration. Close your eyes throughout the practice. First :

△ Inhale and focus on the inner end of the eye (on the side of the nose), while perfectly balancing perception on both sides.

▽ Exhale deeply and shift your attention to the outer edge of both eyes, towards the temples.

This constitutes one cycle. Perform five to ten cycles.

Next, feel and visualize your eyes, imagining them larger, and especially wider, as if they extended all the way to your temples. Combine this movement with eye relaxation as you've learned to do.

If your tensions are high, you may feel stiffness or even pain in your eyes. In this case, perform a series of several cycles, alternating with eye relaxation.

N° 4 – PALMING

Rub your palms together vigorously for a few moments to energize them, then apply them in a dome shape to each of your eyes, without touching them and eliminating the passage of light. Close your eyes, letting them absorb all the vitality of your hands, and concentrate on seeing the darkness and relaxing your eyes and mind.

Repeat the whole process once or twice.

N° 5 – PALMING AND EYE BREATHING ★★★

Part 1:

Resume palming, relax the eyes and begin eye breathing.

△ Inhale: prâna passes through the eyes to the inside of the head.

▽ Exhale: send the prâna back in front of you through the eyeballs.

The first few times, just take a few breaths and make sure your eyes get used to it gradually.

Part 2:

This is a more advanced variant, and should only be performed once you're comfortable with the previous exercise.

Then proceed as follows:

△ Inhale: let the prâna enter your eyes.

▽ Exhale: direct the prâna towards the back of the eyeballs.

Part 3:

△ Inhale: let the prâna enter your eyes.

▽ Exhale: expand the back of the eyeballs towards the back of the head.

Of course, you don't have to do all three steps every time.

N° 6 – PALMING AND THE INNER EYE SPACE ★★★

Perform palming, then :

△ Inhale: enter your eyes and discover their spherical shape.

▽ Exhale: imagine/discover the unlimited inner space of each eye, then of both eyes.

N° 7 – PALMING AND THE SPACE BEHIND THE EYES ★★★

Perform palming, then :

△ Inhale: visualize and feel the spherical shape of the eyes.

▽ Exhale: imagine/visualize the (subtle) space behind the eyes.

In Dr. Bates' eye rehabilitation method, also known as "eye yoga", exercises are performed with accessories. They are also highly effective. These exercises are particularly popular at Sri Aurobindo's ashram in Pondicherry.

We can also add reading or vision with grid glasses. Preferably with pyramid-shaped holes.

> *Eye relaxation training has become indispensable for all mental concentration practices—not least because of the generalization of mental stress and the harmfulness of multiple computer screens. Eye gymnastics create a break in mental tension and restore relaxation and balance to the eyes.*

Prânâyâma:
Preparation for Meditation

V
BREATHING:
OUR FIRST RESOURCE

The basics of prânâyâma

Prâna is life energy or vital force, universal or individual.

The term "prânâyâma" is translated in two different ways.

◊ Either it is considered to be formed from the Sanskrit words "prâna" (vital energy) and "yama", meaning control, and is written prânâyama (control or mastery of prâna).

◊ Or, if it's made up of two words prâna and âyâma, it's written prânâyâma. "Âyâma" means: extension, growth, expansion, amplification, deployment, development. Both translations make sense, but anyone familiar with the nature of prâna will prefer the second. We also prefer the latter interpretation. It should be added that the word is generally transcribed as "prânâyâma" (with three long "a"), which reinforces our choice. It can be translated as the science (or art) of yogic breathing, or simply YOGA BREATHING.

The achievements of the science of yogic breathing (prânâyâma) are many and varied. It can lead us to states of altered consciousness, to trance, in which the breath can stop for long periods, or awaken tremendous energies within us, but we'll remember first and foremost that it is capable of relaxing and balancing us. In fact, as far as we know, there is no more effective way of bringing *balance to* the human psyche and body than *prânâyâma*, which yoga regards as the cornerstone of all higher evolution. In addition, certain rhythms relax, release or expand our *citta*, and relaxation is the first result. Another outcome of *prânâyâma* practice is the mastery *of Prâna. Prâna* is, by its very nature, a balanced force, and therefore also soothing and healing.

> *In the context we have identified for our productivist and technological age, which is highly unbalanced and stressful for our minds and bodies, meditation must integrate energetic and psychological rebalancing. For this, prânâyâma is our most effective and precious tool.*

How do we breathe?

In tense, emotional situations, or when completely absorbed in intellectual activity, the breath becomes shallow, short, irregular and rapid. Inhalation predominates over exhalation, or the breath is blocked. On the other hand, breathing takes place through the top of the lungs, to the detriment of abdominal breathing.

> *Natural breathing is regular, abdominal and deep.*
> *Exhalation should predominate over inhalation.*

Breathing can take place on three different levels: abdominal, thoracic and clavicular.

Natural breathing is complete breathing, incorporating all three stages. But abdominal breathing is the most important of the three. This is the breathing of the young child. It allows maximum air intake with minimum effort, sets the diaphragm in motion, stimulates the solar plexus and massages the abdominal organs. Its action on the diaphragm and solar plexus promotes relaxation. On the other hand, stimulation of the solar plexus encourages the body's metabolism to function properly. It's abdominal breathing that we should be focusing on, as it's the most connected to the body. It's our base, our foundation, our stability.

In yoga, thoracic breathing is linked to emotion, while clavicular breathing is associated with intellectual activity. But that doesn't mean we become smarter by breathing from the top of the chest! In fact, we can see that as soon as there's emotion, belly-breathing stops working, and as soon as there's mental effort or tension, breathing moves to the top of the lungs.

The four beats of breathing

1 – Inspiration

This is the active phase of breathing, the entry of energy. Generally speaking, inspiration connects us with the sense organs and externalization. It predominates during the day and in negative emotions, such as sadness or fear. It encourages activity, action and strength. But it often accompanies muscular or mental tension.

More positively, inspiration is linked to the absorption of vitality. And all the more so as it takes place slowly.

2 – Exhalation

Exhalation is the passive phase of breathing. It represents the release of energy, accompanied by muscular and mental relaxation. It is also associated with the elimination of toxins and used energies, as well as emotions and tensions, all the more so when it is carried out rapidly or strongly, as in the case of purifying breaths or bellows. It can be associated with shouting, singing or violent gestures.

Slow exhalation, on the other hand, speeds up energy exchange and encourages the body's various systems to function optimally.

Exhalation generates calm, peace, rest, openness and receptivity, letting go, relaxation, expansion and joy. It predominates at night and in laughter and tenderness.

Breath-holding

The two retentions of the breath lead to the stability of the inner environment, the citta[1]. They constitute the two most powerful stages of breathing. In ancient texts, prânâyâma was synonymous with Kumbhaka (breath retention).

3 – Holding the breath with full lungs (kumbhaka)

The full-lung retention or suspension of the breath is the highest attainment of inhalation, just as empty-lung retention is for exhalation.

It generates energetic and mental concentration, physical and psychic strength and body warmth. It increases vitality and concentrates prâna.

---

1. Citta is the substance of consciousness.

Kumbhaka accelerates exchanges in the body. But when it is unconscious, it is also sometimes synonymous with blockage and contraction, as in fear.

Thought and emotion are stopped. Full breath retention creates a dynamic position of consciousness, a force for outer life; it generates stability of the inner environment and psyche, and promotes equality of soul. It develops intellectual qualities, optimism, self-confidence and maturity, and encourages psychological fulfillment.

4 – Holding the breath with empty lungs (shunyaka[1])
Retention or suspension on empty lungs leads to relaxation, receptivity and interiorization, contact with the inner being and, like kumbhaka, stabilizes prâna and citta.

Shunyaka eliminates tension and blockages through openness and inner peace. Eliminating blockages enables assimilation and accelerates psychic, energetic and physical exchanges.

It engenders a passive position, a letting go, a sacrifice of personal will. Indeed, we are unable to withstand *shunyaka* if our mind is too active, or if we are drawn into emotion. Empty retention is linked to trust, to letting go of personal willpower, and is predominant in joy, laughter, tenderness and deep interiorization.

Shunyaka leads to contact with the inner self, orienting us towards the inner life and bringing the stability born of peace, withdrawal from action and life, and the disappearance of opposites.

Yoga uses the four beats of the breath and recognizes, as we have seen, an energetic and psychological functionality for each of them. But the most important thing to remember is the importance of exhalation and empty retention for relaxation and internalization.

As part of a yoga of self-transformation and access to transcendence, which goes beyond balance and health, the Indian tradition recognizes the two breath retentions as the two most powerful beats.

1. Shunyaka is neuter.

VI
BREATH
CONTROL

Natural breathing

For many of us, breathing has been disturbed so many times by our emotions that it has become distorted, distorted and imperfect. To correct these defects, we need to learn several things. First of all, the physical zones that have been blocked can be made supple again through specific stretching exercises. For example, we'll stretch the lateral sides of the ribcage if the blockages are at this level. In fact, we'll all benefit from freeing up our breathing by systematically loosening up all areas of the back, the front and sides of the ribcage, the clavicle area and the upper back. Yoga postures (âsanas) serve this function perfectly. To this we add the release of the diaphragm, for which we recommend the practice of *Uddîyâna* bandha, *which* is particularly effective. We describe it in N° 49.

We'll complete our objective with the practice of abdominal breathing and complete breathing, but also in the various breathing practices that emphasize regularity of breath and control of the four beats. It should be noted that it sometimes happens that one or more beats of the breath stubbornly resist all our efforts. This reveals a subconscious trauma.[1] This constitutes a temporary contraindication to prânâyâma until such time as liberating psychotherapy has been undertaken.

---

1. We prefer, with Sri Aurobindo, to use the word "subconscious" rather than "unconscious", which is more precise and more appropriate, since the unconscious assumes that there is no consciousness residing there, which is manifestly inaccurate, even if this limited consciousness has not risen to the surface.

We'll now take a look at some basic yoga breathing techniques.

Abdominal breathing

N° 8 – ABDOMINAL BREATHING ★★★

Lying on your back with one hand on your stomach and the other on your chest, breathe through your belly without moving your ribcage. As you breathe in, your belly inflates and your abdominal muscles rise; as you breathe out, your belly retracts and descends.

△ As you inhale, your belly relaxes and inflates.

▽ As you exhale, it contracts. Check that the belly movement is correct.

Once you've mastered this breathing technique lying down, practice it sitting up. Then practice it slowly throughout the day, as often as possible.

VARIANT: DIAPHRAGM MOVEMENT

Here's an abdominal breathing concentration that amplifies the relaxation effects: visualize and physically feel the movement of the diaphragm as it curves downwards on the inhale and upwards on the exhale.

> *Please note! In yoga, all breathing is done through the nose,*
> *unless otherwise specified for particular techniques.*
> *Prânâyâma is performed on an empty stomach. After the practice,*
> *wait half an hour before eating or making any physical effort.*

Complete breathing

N° 9 – COMPLETE BREATHING ★★★

First and foremost, we need to be aware that breathing is not achieved by voluntarily drawing in air through the nostrils or mouth, but by a suction movement—as in the case of a vacuum pump—created by an expansion of the lung "bag.

The **respiratory muscles** and **diaphragm** synchronize to expand the space in the rib cage:

1 – **From below** (the diaphragm descends, inflating the abdomen)

2 – **Lateral** expansion of the ribcage on the sides, forwards and backwards, in all directions.

3 – **From above,** by raising the clavicles and expanding the upper part of the chest, the clavicular area, especially towards the front, but also, to a lesser extent, in the upper back and laterally, below the armpits.

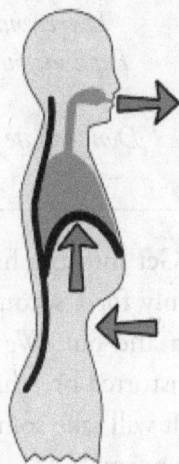

The enlargement of the ribcage, which is integral with the lungs, causes the lungs to expand, creating a **vacuum** that draws air through the nostrils or mouth[1] into the lungs.

From a practical point of view, this is important because the effort will be focused on controlling the chest and stomach muscles and relaxing the nostrils, leading to greater ease of breathing and mental relaxation, and enabling silent breathing.

In a seated position, back straight, abdominal muscles relaxed[2], inhale by first inflating the abdomen, then the ribcage, from bottom to top until the collarbones are lifted – BUT WITHOUT LIFTING OR CONTRACTING THE SHOULDERS – then on exhale, slowly let the collarbones descend[3], then let the chest return to its resting position and finally exhale the rest of the breath by contracting the abdominal muscles.

In this method[4], inspiration is from the bottom up and exhalation from the top down.

---

1. If the glottis passage is open. Note, on the other hand, that if we perform the same movement of ribcage expansion after closing the glottis, the only flexible wall being the diaphragm, it is the diaphragm that is drawn upwards by this thoracic depression – this then draws the belly inwards, as in the Uddîyâna bandha (N° 49).

2. This involves tilting the pelvis forward (anteversion).

3. There's no need to exert any effort, since the ribcage just needs to be lowered!

4. We recommend this method because we learned it in India and practiced it enough to appreciate its consistency and effectiveness. Other methods exist in India.

> *Leave your shoulders relaxed, as well as your neck, jaws and face.*
> *Expand your belly, ribcage and upper lungs as much in the back and*
> *sides as in the front. ·*
> *Don't inflate your belly to the maximum during the inhale, don't try to*
> *inhale to the maximum of your capacity.*

Get into the habit of suspending your breath, full and empty, even if only for a second. This will encourage you to "calm down, not to rush in and out. We need to replace the automatic, unconscious reflexes of distorted breathing with corrected, conscious breathing.

It will take some time[1] to harmonize the movement. This learning time is normal.

Once you've acquired all these reflexes, you can practice the exercises that follow.

As we've seen, in India, the belly is said to be linked to the functioning of the body, the thoracic zone to the emotions and the clavicular zone to the mind. Mastery of the complete breath, integrating the three stages–abdominal, thoracic and clavicular–thus enables us to exert an influence on the whole human being.

Conversely, we would say, with André Van Lysebeth, that our breathing expresses the totality of who we are.

Perfecting the breath
N° 10 – CONTROL OF INSPIRATION, SAHAJ PÛRAKA PRÂNÂYÂMA
△ Inhale very slowly: gradually lengthen the breath to 30 seconds.
▽ Exhale fully, naturally and quietly, passively, without hurrying.
Take about ten breaths. With daily practice, you'll soon reach 30 seconds.

N° 11 – EXHALATION CONTROL, SAHAJ RECHAKA PRÂNÂYÂMA
Proceed in the same way.
△ Inhale deeply and naturally.
▽ Exhale: take control of the exhalation and gradually lengthen the breath to 30 seconds.

1. It can take several months to completely master all the prânâyâma reflexes with their associated retentions and bandhas.

Nº 12 – SPLIT BREATHING, VILOMA PRÂNÂYÂMA

Here's a particular breath in which the inhalation and exhalation are split. Breathe slowly and evenly.

First variant: fractional exhalation

△ Inspiration is normal, but uniform and deep.

▽ Then exhale for 2 seconds, hold for 2 seconds, exhale for 2 seconds, hold for 2 seconds, and so on. You can easily integrate five stages.

Second variant: fractionated inspiration

In this variant, we only split the inspiration.

△ Inhale for 2 seconds, hold for 2 seconds, exhale for 2 seconds, hold for 2 seconds, and so on.

▽ Exhalation is normal.

Third variant: split inhalation and exhalation

Once you've mastered the two splits, train in the same way, splitting both the inhale and exhale.

△ Fractional inspiration.

▽ Fractional exhalation.

VII
THE PRÂNÂYÂMAS OF
RELAXATION

Traditional prânâyâmas

The eight traditional prânâyâmas of yoga are: Ujjâyî, Sûrya bhedana, Bhastrikâ, Plavini, Moorchâ, Shîtalî, Sîtkarî and Bhrâmarî, meditative form of Ujjâyî, N° 19, Bhastrikâ, N° 36, and Bhrâmarî, the Bee, N° 71, are discussed in this book.

Exhalation, a source of relaxation and elimination

N° 13 – DOUBLE EXHALATION (RHYTHM 1:2)

We have already seen that exhalation exerts a relaxing influence. This is why it is favoured in prânâyâma. Remember that lengthening the breath amplifies its effects.

Generally speaking, the exhalation is twice as long as the inhalation. This gives the rhythm 1:2: if you inhale in 4 seconds, you'll exhale in 8.

Sit back and start breathing. Start with 5:10, doubling the exhalation, then gradually increase the rhythm: 5:10; 6:12, 7:14 and so on. The longer you exhale, the deeper the relaxation.

> For a successful long exhalation, remember to start very slowly!

N° 14 – AMPLIFYING EXHALATION, RECHAKA PRÂNÂYÂMA

Here we see some traditional variations with the emphasis on the exhale.

The HA sound on exhale (in a low voice)

△ Normal breathing through the nostrils.

▽ Very slow, long exhalation through the mouth with the HA sound.

Exhaling in Kaki mudrâ

△ Normal breathing through the nostrils.

▽ Exhale very slowly through the mouth in *Kaki mudrâ*.[1]

Exhalation in Sheetalî[2] prânâyâma

△ Normal breathing through the nostrils.

▽ Exhale very slowly through the mouth, pursing the lips or placing the upper lip over the lower. The emphasis is on elimination and purification.

By tightening the passage, internal pressure increases – which is what this exercise is all about.

N° 15 – AMPLIFY EXHALATION ABRUPTLY, SLOW KAPÂLABHÂTI ★★★

The variants of this chapter are known as purification prânâyâmas. The breathing of the Bellows, Kapâlabhâti, in a rapid rhythm, is described further on in N° 29.

Make a **slow** bellows movement with a series of sudden but regular exhalations through the mouth:

First variant:

▽ Powerful exhalation in Kaki mudrâ, with the sound WOOH.

The second, more powerful variant:

▽ Exhale with PPOOH sound.

Practice one or two dozen breaths for each of the two variations.

N° 16 – TRIANGULAR RELAXATION BREATHING (1:1:1) ★★★

This rhythm combines the qualities of balance and relaxation. It equalizes the three beats of the breath: inhalation, *pûraka*, exhalation, *rechaka*,

---

1. Kaki = raven. In Kaki mudrâ, the lips form an O.

2. Sheetali prânâyâma is a summer breath; one of its variants exhales with pursed lips. We'll come back to Sheetali in N° 70 (chapter 11).

and retention on empty lungs (*shunyaka*). Look for uniformity of breath and relaxation of the body.

Once you're familiar with this rhythm, you can visualize a triangle with its point at the top.

△ On the inhale, in 5 seconds, for example, raise the two arms of the triangle towards its apex; hold the breath for one second.

▽ As you exhale, with the same 5-second duration, lower the triangle to the same rhythm as your breathing.

▼ Remain with empty lungs for 5 seconds, while visualizing the base of the triangle. Identify the apex of the triangle with the energy point called *Trikutî*, located in the indentation between the forehead and nose, between the eyebrows.

This breathing, with its emphasis on exhalation and empty retention, is particularly effective for mental relaxation and internalization. In this sense, it is an excellent preparation for meditation.

Inner peace

N° 17 – THE NINE BREATHS

Here we're going to use the relaxing power of exhalation.

Take a series of nine breaths, each with a different concentration.

△ Inhale deeply.

▽ With long, slow exhalations, relax in a dilating motion: the brain (1), shoulders (2), nape of the neck (3), jaws and tongue (4), eyes and temples (5), forehead and skull (6), whole face (7), brain (8), and (9) end this series with the ninth breath, relaxing the mind.

Then remain for a few moments in this feeling of mental relaxation, or start a new cycle.

N° 18 – BRAIN RELAXATION

Preferably close your eyes.

△ Inhale through both nostrils, symmetrically, and raise the subtle breath in a slow, gentle breath to *Trikutî*, the energy center at the top of the nostrils, in the indentation between the nose and the forehead.

▽ Then exhale for a long time in an inner movement of brain relaxation. The sensation starts at *Trikutî* and extends to the whole head. Take about ten breaths in this way.

When you have reached a deep relaxation of the head, stop the exercise and remain still for a few moments, internalized in this pleasant sensation.

N° 19 – UJJÂYÎ PRÂNÂYÂMA[1] ★★★

Ujjâyî is the name of a very special breath in which the glottis is tightened, giving rise to a muffled sound during breathing. With a little practice, you'll not only be able to produce this sound on both the inhale and exhale breaths, but also to modulate it more or less loudly and keep it uniform. This slight training is absolutely essential before moving on to more advanced exercises. This tightening of the glottis is characteristic of the breathing that plays a decisive role in meditation-oriented prânâyâma.

The complete Ujjâyî prânâyâma method corresponds to an advanced prânâyâma, with breath retention, mudrâs-bandhas and concentration. It is outside the scope of this book.

To learn it, pronounce the HA sound for a long time in a low voice as you inhale and exhale. You'll notice that the glottis is closed. Then make the same sound with your mouth closed.

Start practicing the exhalation. Once you've mastered the exhale, add the inhale. Then train to even out the sound and equalize the duration of the 2 beats.

Once you've mastered the technique, you can practice equalizing your inhale and exhale in Ujjâyî, then control your breath so that it flows slowly, deeply and, above all, evenly. With practice, bring the sound down to a minimum. In India, we say that you should be the only one to hear it. Keep concentrating for a few minutes on this sound, which is always the same.

Ujjâyî emphasizes interiorization and relaxation. Practised in this context, it is often associated with the *Khecarî mudrâ*, which consists of placing the tip of the tongue upside down on the upper palate.

Ujjâyî is one of the most extraordinary types of breathing, with multiple effects on the body and psyche. We'll just mention its relaxing effects and

1. The breath of the Victorious.

its ability to help control emotions, particularly fear.

In terms of health, Ujjâyî is effective for calming asthma attacks[1] or irregular heartbeats, especially if practised regularly. In the latter case, the duration of inhalation and exhalation will be equal, and retentions (for the heart), if any, will not exceed 4 seconds.

Ujjâyî is practiced slowly and regularly for relaxation and internalization, with the lowest possible sound.

Emotional management

But if you want to use it to manage emotions, especially powerful ones, you'll need to practice it with a powerful breath, a loud sound, more or less rapidly, striving to balance the duration of the inhale and exhale.

VARIANT 1: THE SOUND OF THE WAVE ON THE SAND

The sound the waves make as they roll over the sand follows a gradually increasing and decreasing intensity curve. This sound is very relaxing. In this variation, imitate the sound of one wave as you inhale and another as you exhale, using the characteristic *Ujjâyî* sound. If you want to accentuate the effect, plug your ears.

VARIANT 2: UJJÂYÎ, WITH THE KHECARÎ MUDRÂ[2] ★★★

Adopt a comfortable posture, then begin the Ujjâyî breath, as learned in N° 19. Concentrate on the regularity and uniformity of the sound, then equalize the duration of the four beats of the breath. Finally, turn your tongue over onto the upper palate, as high as possible, without excess.

Start by applying the *Khecarî mudrâ* only on the inhale and exhale, and relax your tongue on both retentions, until your tongue muscles get used to it. You can then hold it in all four strokes.

△ Inhale in Ujjâyî, with *Khecarî mudrâ*, in 8 seconds.

▲ Hold the *Khecarî* and add *Mûla bandha* to the kumbhaka in 8 seconds.

▽ Exhale into Ujjâyî with *Khecarî mudrâ* in 8 seconds.

1. Only if you have mastered this prânâyama before.

2. The Khecarî mudrâ in its simplest form consists of turning the tip of the tongue towards the upper palate. It is described in exercise 40.

▾ Hold the empty breath with *Khecarî mudrâ* and *Mûla bandha* in 8 seconds.

If you're looking for interiorization and inner calm, it's always a good idea to practice your breathing in Ujjâyî. Khecarî *mudrâ* amplifies the effects. The practice of Ujjâyî concentrates energies in Sushumnâ, the central channel.

N° 20 – UJJÂYÎ IN JÂLANDHARA BANDHA ★★★

In this deeper exercise, we practice Ujjâyî in the meditation position, combining it with Khecharî mudrâ and half a Jâlandhara bandha[1], with retentions of one to two seconds, leaving the glottis semi-open.

Practice ten or so breaths, then relax and go inward.

---

1. Jâlandhara bandha, the throat bandha: exercise N° 80.

VIII
BREATHING FOR
BALANCING

Energy and psychic balancing

In yoga, the human being is influenced by two antagonistic and complementary forces, which circulate in two different *nâdîs*, located respectively to the left and right of the spinal column, and which are called *Idâ* and *Pingalâ*.

Idâ is lunar and oriented towards psychic life; it is linked to the left nostril, the left hemicorpus and the right brain.

Pingalâ is solar and action-oriented; it corresponds to the right nostril, the right hemisphere and the left hemisphere of the brain. Generally speaking, these two internal energies alternate, with one predominating over the other on a fairly regular basis.

But if, for a short time, these two forces are balanced, *prâna* awakens in the central *nâdî* called **Sushumnâ**[1], and the human being moves to a higher, more subtle, spiritual energy level, conducive to balance and meditation, in a state free of all tensions. This is why yogis have created practices to balance these two *nâdîs*.

This can be achieved by concentrating on balancing either the two hemispheres, or the two nostrils, or the two cerebral hemispheres. However, internal energy balancing can also be achieved by distributing *prâna* between the posterior and anterior parts of the body, or between the upper and lower parts of the body. This is particularly apparent in the "Kirlian

1. *Sushumnâ* is the most important *nâdî*. It is located in the pranic body and corresponds to the spinal cord.

photograph, which shows an imprint around the hands or feet (cf. *Soothe your mind*, pp. 144 & 145).

We could say that if the two *nâdîs Idâ* and *Pingalâ* are the expression of dualities in man, *Sushumnâ* is the channel of superior balance and transcendence.

However, Ida / Pingala rebalancing is the best, most universally accessible method yoga has to offer for psychological rebalancing. And psychological balance takes precedence over any internalization or spiritual discipline.

Here's a chart[1] showing the differences between *Idâ* and *Pingalâ*.

Idâ	Pingalâ
negative	positive
female	male
left	right
yin	yang
moon	sun
cold	hot
intuition	logic
desire	action
subconscious	conscious
internal	external
night	day
liabilities	dynamics
parasympathetic	friendly
blue	red
right hemisphere	left hemisphere (brain)
left hemisphere	right hemisphere
citta	prâna

The Idâ and Pingalâ nâdîs

Three main energy channels distribute prâna to the body. These are Sushumnâ at the center of the spine, Idâ to the left of the spine and linked to the left side of the body, and Pingalâ to the right and linked to the right side of the body.

We present three representations here.

The first represents the nâdis in a straight line.

1. This painting is inspired by Swami Satyananda's book: *Âsanas, prânâyâma, mudrâs et bandhas*, Satyananda Éditions.

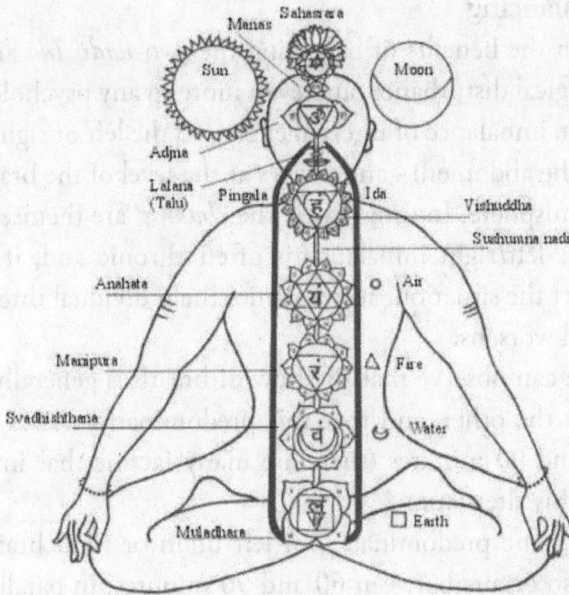

The other representations are pictured in a spiral pattern. The one on the left gives a better view of the chakras, but in Indian teaching, the two nâdîs cross at each chakra (figure on the right).

Rectilinear or spiral representations are fair and not antagonistic. It all depends on practice.

Simply remember that Idâ is linked to the left and Pingalâ nâdi is connected to the right side of the body.

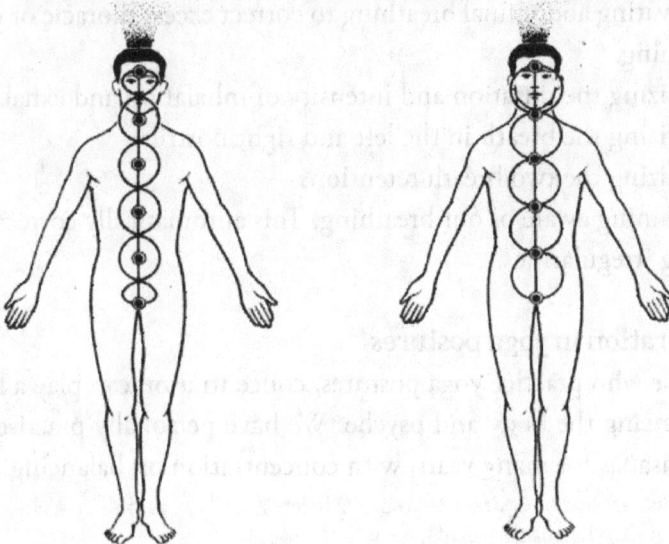

Left/right balancing

We have seen the benefits of balancing the two *nâdîs Idâ* and *Pingalâ*. Any psychological disturbance, and even more so any psychological trauma, leads to an imbalance of internal energy to the left or right, either locally (e.g. in the abdomen) – and always at the level of the brain – or over the whole hemisphere. In some cases, the *chakras*[1] are themselves shifted sideways. This left/right imbalance is often chronic and, if nothing is done to correct the situation, accompanies the individual throughout his or her life and worsens.

Similarly, we can observe that the flow of breath is generally greater in one nostril or the other, and that this predominance varies on average between 60 and 90 minutes (there are many factors that influence the regularity of this alternation).

We find the same predominance of left brain or right brain, and the alternation also occurs between 60 and 90 minutes, in parallel with the nostrils. Last but not least, sleep is divided into 90-minute periods.

The slightest emotion instantly disturbs our breathing, but controlling the breath stabilizes the mind. So if we want to turn things around and regain calm, concentration and balance, we need to control our breathing.

This energetic and psychological rebalancing can be achieved in five different ways:

By reactivating abdominal breathing to correct excess thoracic or clavicular breathing.

En equalizing the duration and intensity of inhalation and exhalation

En equalizing the breath in the left and right nostrils.

En equalizing the two breath retentions

Eby remaining aware of our breathing. This automatically corrects many breathing irregularities.

Concentration in yoga postures

For those who practice yoga postures, concentration can play a key role in rebalancing the body and psyche. We have personally practised – and taught – âsanas for many years, with concentration on balancing the two

1. The *chakras* are the control centers for internal energy and the psyche. They are also gateways to the subtle worlds.

hemispheres or on the whole body, felt as a totality. As well as bringing about good internalization, they generate the stability and balance we all need, and maintain the body's health. In the same vein, we can also add concentration on the equalization of inhalation and exhalation in the static part of the postures. In this way, we combine the beneficial effects of posture, prânâyâma and meditation.

N° 21 – ALTERNATE BREATHING, NÂDÎ SHODANA PRÂNÂYÂMA[1] ★★★

In India, this prânâyâma is considered one of the most important breathing practices. This chapter covers the first stages. The higher degrees will be described in chapter 13, along with breath retention.

In this breathing exercise, we will equalize the breath in both nostrils to restore *prâna* balance and remove energy blockages. In India, this breathing is highly recommended for its capacity to purify the nâdîs[2], and is practiced for several months before tackling *prânâyâmas* with breath retention.

In a seated position, breathing fully, back straight, alternately block one nostril with the thumb and the other with the ring and little fingers together. The middle two fingers are folded over the palm or placed on the forehead.

△ Inhale through the left nostril.

▽ Exhale through the right nostril.

△ Inhale through the right nostril.

▽ Exhale through the left nostril.

This constitutes a cycle.

Practice five to ten cycles with the right hand and as many cycles with the left, equalizing the duration of inhalation and exhalation and gradually lengthening the breath. The slower and more regular the breath, the greater the benefits.

Relax your nostrils as you inhale, and keep your face and shoulders relaxed at all times. We'll look at the next steps later.

---

1. Nâdîshodana means: purification of the nâdîs.
2. Nâdîs are to the prânic body what nerves and veins are to the physical body.

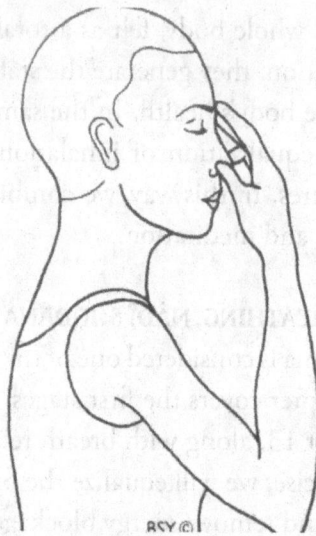

Nâdî Shodana

N° 22 – NÂDÎ SHUDDHI PRÂNÂYÂMA, rectangular alternate breathing (2 : 1 : 2 : 1) ★★★

Nâdî shuddhi and Nâdî shodana are similar prânâyâmas, with alternate left and right breathing. Traditionally, Nâdî Shodana is a superior prânâyâma, for balancing Ida and Pingala and purifying the nâdîs. The proportion between the four beats varies.

In Nâdî Shuddhi, inhalation and exhalation are balanced, as are the two retentions. This is a remarkable balancing prânâyâma.

For example, 8 : 4 : 8 : 4.

△ Inhale through the left nostril in 8 seconds.

▲ Hold your breath for 4 seconds.

▽ Exhale through the right nostril in 8 seconds.

▼ Hold your breath for 4 seconds.

△ Inhale through the right nostril in 8 seconds.

▲ Hold your breath for 4 seconds.

▽ Exhale through the left nostril in 8 seconds.

▼ Hold your breath for 4 seconds.

This constitutes a cycle. Practice 5 to 10 cycles.

NÂDÎ SHUDDHI SUPERIOR
Increase the duration
Work your way up to 16 : 8 : 16 : 8.

VARIANT – NÂDÎ SHUDDHI PRÂNÂYÂMA AND COLOURED PRÂNA
Rhythm (2 : 1 : 2 : 1)
For example, here 8 : 4 8 : 4 or 10 : 5 : 10 : 5.
- △▲ Inhale through left nostril and kumbhaka, visualizing light pink prâna.
- ▽▼ Exhale through the right nostril and shunyaka with the visualization of light-blue prâna.
- △▲ Inhale through the right nostril and kumbhaka with the visualization of pink prâna.
- ▽▼ Exhale through left nostril and shunyaka with visualization of blue prâna.

N° 23: ANULOMA VILOMA, PSYCHIC ALTERNATE BREATHING ★★★
This alternating breathing is practiced without hands, using imagination and concentration alone.
- △▽ Inhale through the left nostril and exhale through the right.
- △▽ Inhale through the right nostril and exhale through the left.

This forms a cycle. Practice a minimum of 10 cycles. Equalize the inhale and exhale and breathe evenly.

VARIANT: WITH PrânaVA
Chant the AUM mentally on the inhale and exhale.

(N° 71) – BEE BREATHING AND BALANCE
Here, vibrate the sound in one ear only, plugging it with your finger, alternating left and right with each exhalation. Finish by balancing both sides for five breaths.

The five prânas
The subtle physiology of yoga describes 10 forms of prâna in the body. Of these, five are important:

Prâna vâyu, located in the chest, is responsible for incoming energy, both physical and energetic. It is managed by the Heart chakra, Anâhata, and has an ascending movement.

Samâna vâyu, in the solar plexus and stomach area, represents the energy of digestion and assimilation; it depends on the Manipûra chakra.

Apâna vâyu is located in the pelvis and legs; it is the energy of elimination. It is managed by the base chakra, Mûlâdhâra, and moves downwards.

Udâna vâyu is located in the throat and head; it depends on the Vishuddha chakra and deals with expression and basic mental energies. Its movement is upward.

Vyâna vâyu is controlled by Swâddhisthâna, in the pelvis, but its action extends to the whole physical body: for it manages all circulation in the subtle physical body.

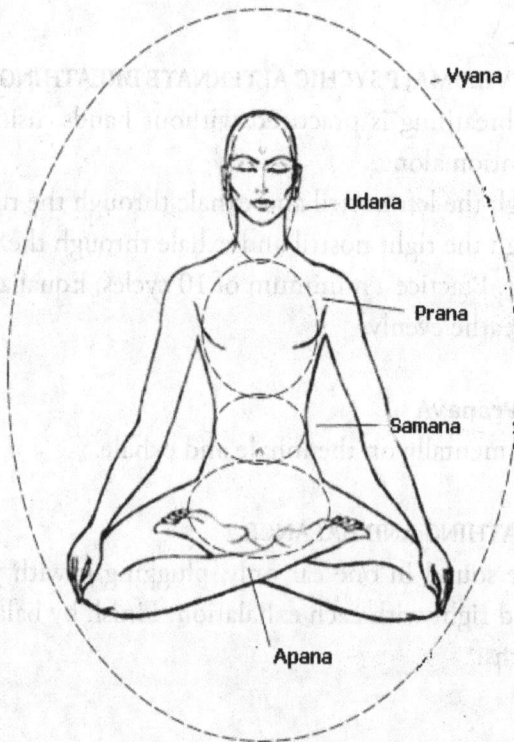

The 5 prânas

The power of rhythm

Equalizing inhalation and exhalation equalizes and rebalances Prâna and Apâna, the energy that flows in and the energy that flows out.

N° 24 – TRIANGULAR BREATHING FOR CONCENTRATION (1 : 1 : 1) ★★★

All three beats are equal.

△ Inhale, for example, in 8 seconds.

▲ Hold your breath for 8 seconds.

▽ Exhale in 8 seconds.

This gives 8 : 8 : 8.

Maintain this rhythm for about ten breaths, then close your eyes and keep your concentration on the passage of the breath through your nostrils for a few moments.

N° 25 – SÂVITRÎ PRÂNÂYÂMA, RECTANGULAR BREATHING (2 : 1 : 2 : 1) ★★★

Sâvitrî prânâyâma[1] introduces the four beats of breathing and equates them two by two. The two movements of inhalation and exhalation, through the two nostrils, will therefore be equal, as will the two retentions, the duration of which will extend over half of the inhalation and exhalation. This gives 2 : 1 : 2 : 1.

△ Inhale, for example, in 8 seconds.

▲ Hold your breath for four seconds.

▽ Exhale in 8 seconds.

▼ Remain for 4 seconds on empty lungs.

This gives 8 : 4 : 8 : 4.

Gradually increase the duration of the four beats as your ease of breathing increases.

VARIANT: RECTANGLE VISUALIZATION

In synchrony with the breath, visualize a rectangle that is taller than it is wide, with the sides running clockwise.

△ As you inhale, you raise your left side.

▲ Traverse the upper side in full-lung retention (*kumbhaka*).

1. *Sâvitrî* is one of the names of the sun in Hindu mythology.

▽ Lower your right side as you exhale.

▼ And traverse the lower base in empty-lung retention (*shunyaka*).

N° 26 – SAMAVRITTI PRÂNÂYÂMA, SQUARE BREATHING (1 : 1 : 1 : 1) ★★★

In this prânâyâma, the four beats of the breath are equalized. Concentrate on the regularity of the breath and progress day by day to gradually increase the length of the breath.

△ Inhale, for example, in 6 seconds.

▲ Hold your breath for 6 seconds.

▽ Exhale in 6 seconds.

▼ Remain on empty lungs for 6 seconds.

VARIANT: ROUNDED CORNERS

In the same way, you can visualize a square. Then round off the four corners. As you progress in your physical and mental relaxation, this rhythm will lengthen, and your internalization and relaxation will deepen.

N° 27 – SHERPA PRÂNÂYÂMA (x : 1 : x : 1) ★★★

This breathing, which is practiced in the exercise of walking, synchronizes the breath with the steps.

△ Inhale for 4 steps.

▲ Hold your breath for one step.

▽ Exhale over 4 steps.

▼ Hold your breath on one step.

Here, the rhythm is 4 : 1 : 4 : 1. The time of the 2 suspensions is always equal to one step. But the inspiratory and expiratory times may vary, depending on your ability and the difficulty of the terrain, whether you're going uphill or downhill. Choose the most suitable rhythm and, if you feel comfortable, lengthen it.

If the terrain is very difficult, continue to equalize the inhales and exhales, but eliminate the suspensions.

This prânâyâma will considerably increase your vitality and endurance.

If you want to go further, you can add concentrations. The most popular are:

Concentration on the whole body, like a block (particularly re-balancing).

Equalization of the 2 hemispheres (therapeutic, it's a classic of deep energetic and psychological balancing).

Concentration on the solar plexus (for vitality).

Concentration on the base chakra, Mûlâdhâra, should be reserved for advanced yoga practitioners. It can be replaced, without reservation, by concentration on the pelvis and legs, or on the feet's relationship with the Earth.

For those who have mastered prâna **perception**:

The perception of prâna in the stomach area (for vitality).

The perception of prâna in the whole body (pranic body).

Communion with the environment through prâna.[1]

In this way, your walk will become therapeutic and regenerative, reinforcing its wellness dimension.

Learn to count without counting

Repetitive mental counting with numbers clutters the mind and can give the unpleasant impression of a mechanical mind. Prânâyâma seeks mental calm, vigilance and inner freedom. Is counting compulsory? And if so, how can we count in a less intrusive way?

In fact, it's important to measure the rhythms of the different breathing beats, otherwise you risk taking away from the rhythm itself and all its benefits. On the other hand, it provides benchmarks against which we can measure our progress.

But we can bring more subtlety to it and free the mind first by doing away with counting with numbers. Indian texts advocate following the rhythm of the heartbeat, but this doesn't necessarily eliminate numbers, and we observe that the rhythm changes according to whether we're in one or the other of the breathing times. It will tend to be faster during kumbhaka and effort, which is inevitable in learning and progress.

Some people recommend repeating a mantra as a measure. Either the mantra AUM, which is repeated to measure time, or a mantra with several syllables, where each syllable counts as a measure[2] of one second. This is a good method.

---

1. Obviously, if the environment is naturally rich in prâna (forest, mountains, seaside...)

2. In Sanskrit, measure = mâtrâ.

What we can do is get used to counting in groups of numbers, without mentally reciting the numbers, which will form the basic measure, which we then repeat according to the length of the cycles. For example, in the rhythm 5 : 10 : 5 : 10, the unit will be five bars, and we can replace the numbers with a sound, like the sound of a metronome, or with 5 AUM or a five-syllable mantra, if you have one.

In this way, we can quickly create a rhythm and direct the measure of our cycles without having to think about it. The sound of the rhythm remains, but the numbers that made it sound disappear. In this way, we can easily go as far as the rhythm of 6. We are perfectly capable of following the rhythm by repeating this unit (here made up of six bars) automatically, against a background of silence. In the cycle 12 : 48 : 24, for example, we repeat our basic measure (here of 6 units) 2 times – 8 times – 4 times. By the way, there's nothing to stop us using the sound of a mechanical alarm clock or metronome to check the rhythm from time to time.

As for the number of cycles covered, with the hands resting on the thighs, we can count with the fingers by applying pressure to the thigh. Some prefer to count the cycles with the thumb in contact with each phalanx, which gives us 12 measurements. Ten or twelve cycles is already good practice.

Finally, you can use a mala[1] and place rubber bands or woollen threads in places corresponding to the rhythm of the day.

However, my preferred method of counting cycles is by visualizing the numbers.

---

1. The mala is an Indian rosary. You can find them in Buddhist centers or, of course, on the Internet.

IX
PRÂNÂYÂMAS
FOR DYNAMIZATION
AND PURIFICATION

Is prânâyâma dangerous?

Prânâyâma is the art of using the breath to receive all the benefits linked to the vital force, Prâna. In this sense, it is a discipline for perfecting and fulfilling the human being, for rebalancing and amplifying his or her capacities. It's not a recent discipline, following fashions like many Western fitness methods. It's a serious, age-old discipline that's never stopped improving.

It's true that Indian yoga is in decline, as is civilization as a whole, and modernity has changed the minds of India's youth, who tend to turn their backs on their age-old tradition.

Prânâyâma is no exception to the rule, and prânâyâma masters – accomplished yogis in their art and science – have become rare. They practiced from five to ten hours a day, achieving superhuman states of consciousness and energy, of which the Kewala kumbhaka[1] is the best-known expression. However, they have left us all the keys to practising it safely, especially if we avoid ambition and remain attached to the culture of common sense.

Clearly, prânâyâma cannot be used as a method of spiritual liberation without the guidance and presence of an accomplished master. The same

1. Kewala kumbhaka is breath-holding for very long periods of time, combined with very advanced states of meditation, without any effort. Could this be the dream of every freedivers?

applies to the traditional methods of Hatha Yoga and Kundalinî Yoga, which are very similar.

But if Western students confine themselves to the basic objectives – and the most motivated rarely exceed one hour's practice – all they need to do is learn the technical gestures, which they can receive from the few teachers who have themselves received them from India. A sensible, healthy, low-toxicity diet, a life free of excess, reasonable stress and a calm environment are all necessary. The electromagnetic environment must also be taken into account and rebalanced.[1]

In fact, the main difficulties that can arise are linked to overdynamization. Overdynamization of the citta and consciousness generates an influx of thoughts and images and can bring emotionality, exaltation, excitement and passion into the mind. This can lead to confusion, intolerance, exclusivism and fanaticism.

The overdynamization of prâna and vitality will stimulate and amplify our impulses, desires, tendencies and mental or vital predispositions, the most common form of expression of which is emotional amplification.

On the physical level, if we're not suffering from any serious disorders, simple dynamization will reduce all our symptoms and therefore tend to improve our health, but overdynamization can lead in the early stages to fever or various intestinal or other symptoms, generally harmless if we correct the excesses.

The solution is to slow down our practice for a day or two, but generally speaking, we need to include peace, balance and stability in our personal development, and focus on the techniques that generate them.

Apart from these considerations, prânâyâma can be started at any age, even advanced, but is not recommended before puberty, with the obvious exception of all the basic breathing exercises, which are beneficial to all and at all ages.

> *The golden rules of yoga practice are self-observation, progressiveness, adaptation and constant concentration on the body's sensations.*

1. There are various systems available, and I've designed one myself. The most efficient is the Keshe Magrav connected to the home's electricity. However, with the advent of the Linky smart meter and 5G, everything is getting more complicated.

Dynamization and purification

(N° 24) – KUMBHAKA TRIANGULAR BREATHING AT THE SOLAR PLEXUS
★★★

Adjust your position for prânâyâma and begin triangular breathing with kumbhaka.

△ Inhale in 8 seconds, for example.

▼ Kumbhaka in 8 seconds: concentration on prâna at the solar plexus + 1/2 *Mûla bandha*.

▽ Exhale in 8 seconds.

Practice for a minimum of 10 breaths, then prolong the concentration on prâna in the body without worrying about breathing.

N° 28 – PRÂNA KUMBHAKA, PRÂNIC RECHARGING ★★★

△ Inhale the prâna at Trikutî in 8 seconds, for example, and simultaneously transport it to the solar plexus.

▼ Kumbhaka in 8 seconds: concentration on prâna at the solar plexus + 1/2 *Mûla bandha*.

▽ Exhaling for 8 seconds, concentrate and visualize the expansion of prâna in Trikutî if you wish to revitalize yourself in a general way. Or send the prâna to a deficient area or organ of the body.

Once the revitalization is complete, continue to concentrate on the prâna and its well-being.

N° 29 – KÂPÂLABHÂTI, THE BELLOWS[1] ★★★

This breathing is essential in prânâyâma. It involves hyperventilation through the abdomen alone (abdominal breathing).

It is characterized by its speed of execution, its exclusive concentration on exhalation, combined with contraction of the abdomen.

In a seated position, with your back straight and your girdle relaxed, suddenly contract your abdominal muscles as you exhale, then immediately release your stomach. Continue with successive, progressively faster contractions until you reach a rhythm of around one contraction per second.

The effort should be placed solely on the exhalation in the contraction,

---

1. *Kapâla*: head, forehead; *bhâti*: to make shine, to radiate. The breath that makes the skull shine.

followed immediately by relaxation of the abdominal strap, resulting in a natural, spontaneous inhalation. Make sure you completely relax the abdominal muscles after each exhalation, if you want the exercise to last.

To begin with, practice *Kapâlabhâti* at the rate of one breath per second, emphasizing the amplitude and therefore the strength of the exhalation. Avoid excess, however, and remember to relax your shoulders and head. Then gradually increase the speed to an average of one or two breaths per second.

Open your glottis: don't practice *Kapâlabhâti* with the muffled sound of *Ujjâyî*. Let's leave that to experienced practitioners of the higher prânâyâma.

Achieve a harmonious compromise between amplitude and speed, without ever sacrificing physical and mental relaxation. Concentrate on the exhalation.

Start with a series of 20 to 30 breaths. Follow with a normal full inhalation and exhalation, and stay on empty lungs (*shunyaka*) for as long as is comfortable. Never exceed your current capacity, as this will result in breathlessness and mental tension. Later, you can replace empty retention by full retention (kumbhaka) with the two bandhas. We'll look at this later.

You can then practice up to three successive series.

Gradually, through regular practice, build up to 50 to 100 breaths, always followed by empty retention and relaxation/concentration.

Physiologically, *Shunyaka* restores the right balance between oxygen and carbon dioxide; energetically and psychologically, it brings relaxation and interiorization.

Practice should bring you interiorization and concentration. Your mind should feel energized and relaxed. Once you've mastered the practice, focus on mental calmness in empty suspension, *Shunyaka* and after retention.

Don't hesitate to be corrected by a competent yoga teacher.

This *prânâyâma* must be performed on an empty stomach.

Kapâlabhâti stimulates and purifies the most advanced (frontal) part of the brain. In just a few minutes, it brings mental calm and a feeling of emptiness, clarity and enlargement in the head space. All this makes it a remarkable exercise for mental calm.

Contraindications:

This exercise, and the two following variations, are contraindicated for people with lung or heart disease. *Kapâlabhâti* is, however, excellent for asthma sufferers.

Kapâlabhâti practice is therefore followed by empty-lung retention. This is all the more interesting as hyperventilation enables you to hold *shunyaka* for a long time, and thus receive all its benefits, especially on the mental level.

In the beginning, empty retention, *shunyaka*, can bring anguish linked to the fear of suffocation. This is of course unfounded, and to the best of our knowledge, empty retention presents no danger unless accompanied by *Uddîyâna bandha*. Regular learning leads to rapid progress, and retention can last a minute or more. During retention, it is therefore very important to relax the mind and the head area (forehead, eyes, jaws, tongue, nape of the neck, shoulders), then learn to remain motionless internally and receptive to the effects of the practice.

Now, if despite all your efforts, empty-lung retention continues to bring you anguish and great difficulty in its execution, even for short durations, this would express past traumas; don't persist any longer and adopt full-lung retention by maintaining it moderately.

We'll see later that *Shunyaka* is a privileged moment for concentration.

In higher prânâyâma practices, vacuum retention is associated with *Mûla bandha* and *Uddîyâna bandha*. This considerably amplifies their power. Similarly, we can adopt one or other of the retentions that follow the Bellows, in which case we use the bandhas. We'll look at the practice in chapter 10 on mudras and bandhas.

N° 30 – BREATHING THE FOUR FACES: BRAHMA OR CATURMUKHI PRÂNÂYÂMA[1]

This breathing is identical to *Kapâlabhâti*, turning the head to the left, then to the right, then up, then down, with a bellows on each exhalation. It is practised more slowly and for much less time than Kapâlabhâti. About ten cycles of four movements are sufficient, and empty retention is not necessary. Then enjoy the peace and mental stability associated with the breathing calm that follows hyperventilation.

1. *Brahma* is a four-headed Hindu deity, and *caturmukhi* means "four-faced".

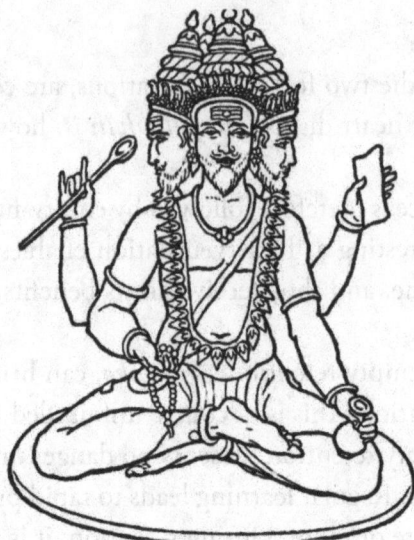

Brahma

N° 31 – CLAVICULAR KAPÂLABHÂTI

This breathing unblocks clavicular breathing.

Here, hyperventilation is achieved not through the belly, but through the top of the lungs. The benefits of this exercise are obvious, as it removes mental tension accumulated in the upper back, chest and shoulders. There are several variations.

Sitting with your back straight, place your hands on your thighs, raise your shoulders by stretching your arms (passive inhalation) and drop them suddenly, accompanying this movement with a voluntary exhalation. Synchronize the practice of the Bellows with this movement of the shoulders.

Practice without interruption for twenty to thirty breaths, then suspend the breath, empty, without forcing, concentrating on mental relaxation.

This breathing is an excellent preparation for prânâyâmas, where the breath is held with full lungs.

VARIANT: WITH ELBOWS

This breathing amplifies thoracic breathing.

You can also perform the sudden exhalation by moving your arms with clenched fists, positioned at chest level, without touching it, and elbows raised (on the inhale). Exhale as you rapidly lower your elbows. Execute a rapid succession of upward and downward movements, synchronizing the exhale with the downward movement. There's also a more advanced variant, in which inhalation and exhalation are equally synchronized with the elbow movements. This latter variant amplifies thoracic breathing the most.

> *All bellows exercises, Kapalabhati, beyond 30 breaths, must*
> *be followed by breath suspension and mental relaxation.*

The following two variants are effective rebalancing practices.

N° 32 – ALTERNATING KAPÂLABHÂTI 1

Place the index and middle fingers of the right hand on the forehead and use the other fingers to block the nostrils. Use the ring and little fingers for the left nostril and the thumb for the right. If you use the left hand, the fingers will be reversed.
△ Inhale through both nostrils.
▽ Exhale with one nostril, alternating L or R.
Continue in this way.
Take about 50 breaths. This variant is easier than the next.

VARIANT – ALTERNATING KÂPÂLABHÂTI 2

Block nostrils with fingers, in the same way.
△ Inhale through the left nostril.
▽ Exhale through the right nostril.
△ Inhale through the right nostril.
▽ Exhale through the left nostril, and so on.

N° 33 – KÂPÂLABHÂTI AND THE SKULL

With head erect and balanced, gazing 1.50 m ahead, practice Kâpâlabhâti, concentrating on the top of the skull.

N° 34 – KÂPÂLABHÂTI, CHIN UP

With your head tilted back and your chin raised as high as possible, without compressing the nape of your neck, practice the Bellows, concentrating on the top of your skull.

Start cautiously with about ten exhalations and observe yourself. Open your glottis wide. Watch out for dizziness! Don't insist if you have difficulty. Totally contraindicated for people with heart problems.

Nº 35 – KÂPÂLABHÂTI, CHIN DOWN

Close your eyes, lower your head until you touch your throat with your chin in the Jâlandhara bandha, concentrate on the back of your neck, then begin the Kapâlabhâti practice.

Practice one or more series of 30 breaths, followed by passive concentration. Develop your sensitivity to the psychic and pranic changes that are bound to occur.

Like its predecessors, this prânâyâma purifies certain prânic areas of the body, unblocking energy channels and improving prâna circulation.

Nº 36 – BHASTRIKÂ PRÂNÂYÂMA (abdomen) ★★★

Here's another breath of the Bellows, which can be tackled after learning Kapâlabhâti.

Bhastrikâ, literally forge bellows, is more powerful than Kapâlabhâti. Here, we describe only the gentle form, practiced with the abdomen only. The more advanced forms, called Mahâbhastrikâ, are practiced with full breathing. They are not recommended without long-standing Kapâlabhâti practice and the supervision of a competent teacher.

With your back straight, arch your back slightly. Add *Mûla bandha*, if necessary, for the duration of the exercise. (*Mûla bandha*[1] can often occur spontaneously).

Breathing will be through the belly only.

△ As you inhale, expand your belly.

▽ As you exhale, contract it.

Equalize the duration of the inhalation and exhalation, and gradually accelerate the breath while concentrating on the uniformity of the breath. This is what distinguishes it from Kapâlabhâti, in which concentration was exclusively on the exhalation.

1. The gesture consists of tightening the sphincters of the anus, as if to close (seal) the passage.

Adopt a rhythm of about one breath per second, a little slower than Kapâlabhâti. Don't exceed fifty breaths at first.

After the Bhastrikâ, breath retention is traditionally a kumbhaka with *Mûla bandha and Jâlandhara bandha*. We'll take a closer look at kumbhaka with these bandhas in Chapter 12. In the meantime, you can practice moderate kumbhakas with *Mûla bandha*.

> *Don't miss the concentrations after the kumbhaka.*
> *They are our reward.*

X
BREATHING AND MUDRÂS-BANDHAS

Mudras and bandhas

Mudras[1] are gestures or positions of the hands, eyes, different parts of the body or the whole body, which modify internal energy and the state of consciousness. They are abundant in oriental dance and widely used in yoga.

Bandhas are muscular contractions, often associated with body positions, whose aim is also to manipulate internal energy (*prâna*) and the substance of consciousness (*citta*). A *bandha* often combines a particular position, a muscular contraction that may be accompanied by an energetic contraction, breath retention and concentration.

Mudras and *bandhas* are often associated because they are often combined in the same practice.

Mudras and bandhas for concentration and interiorization
N° 37 – MUNI MUDRÂ, THE MUDRÂ OF SERENITY[2] ★★★

Muni mudrâ involves slowly lifting the eyebrows upwards and towards the temples, without tensing the forehead. In particular, this mudrâ relaxes the area at the base of the forehead, between the eyebrows. It can be combined with *Bhoochari mudrâ[3]*, with eyes open, but is usually performed with eyes closed.

1. Mudrâ : female.
2. Muni: the Awakened One, the Wise One.
3. Bhoochari mudrâ : see below.

Muni mudrâ instantly brings a sensation of widening, dilation, aeration and luminosity. A sense of release emerges from the mind, an opening of the entire forehead space, as if our gaze were widening upwards. With practice, a gentle joy and bliss invade the inner space of the head. This mudra is often used in meditation.

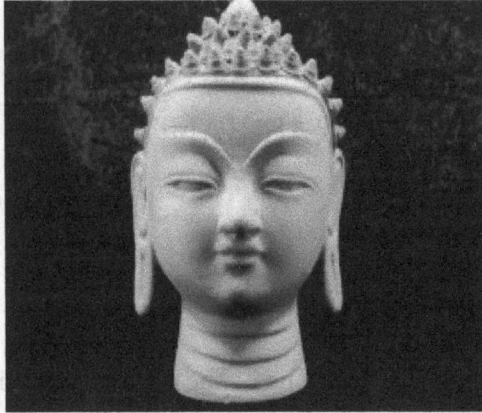

Muni mudrâ

N° 38 – JNÂNA MUDRÂ, THE MUDRÂ OF KNOWLEDGE ★★★

The junction of thumb and forefinger symbolizes the junction of the individual and the universe, or the individual Divine and the cosmic Divine. There are several variations, with different names. The hand can be oriented upwards or downwards, and the thumb can also be placed on the index finger nail.

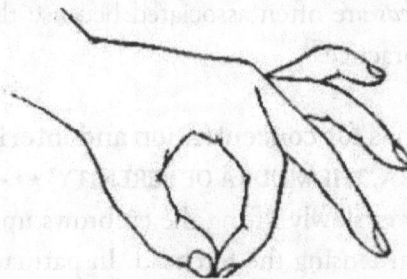

Jnâna mudrâ

This mudrâ reinforces the power of meditation poses by redirecting prâna to the upper body.

N° 39 – BHOOCHARI MUDRÂ, THE MUDRÂ OF EMPTINESS VARIATION 1:
The empty point ★★★

Through the eyes, we act on the mind. Place your hand horizontally, palm down, fingers together against your face, between the nose and upper lip, and focus your gaze on the little finger for a few moments. Then remove your hand and continue to look at the same spot in the space in front of you, concentrating on the void.

VARIATION 2: empty space

Stretch your arm out in front of you, close your hand and raise your thumb. Then concentrate for a few moments on the thumbnail and remove your hand. Then keep your mind on the perception of this point in the void in front of you and expand your visual perception to the whole space in front of you, as large as possible, without hanging your gaze on any object.

Keep your mind firmly on empty space, on the sensation and representation of emptiness. Under no circumstances should you allow your visual awareness to enter the *tamas*[1]. Indeed, there's a big difference between these conscious exercises and staring into space. In both cases, the mind relaxes, but gazing into the void leads the mind into a state of unconsciousness and inertia, whereas *Bhoochari mudrâ* intensifies vigilance. *Bhoochari mudrâ* is also a meditation aid.

N° 40 – KHECARÎ MUDRÂ ★★★

Khecarî mudrâ is an advanced Hatha Yoga mudrâ in which the tongue is turned back against the palate and gradually lengthened so that it can be inserted into the nasal cavity, triggering the onset of trance and supranormal abilities. But there's a simpler form in which the tip of the tongue is simply turned over to touch the soft part of the palate (also known as the "false palate"), which reinforces the effects of prânâyâma Ujjâyî. Ujjâyî tends to dry out the throat, while Khecarî stimulates saliva production. All the more reason to combine them. The Khecarî mudrâ in its simple form is certainly a meditation mudrâ, since it stimulates the Sushumnâ nâdî.

---

1. *Tamas* is one of nature's three essential psychological qualities, synonymous with torpor, inertia and unconsciousness.

N° 41 – INTRODUCTION TO SHÂMBAVÎ, BHOOCHARI AND NASIKÂGRA MUDRÂS

In Nasikâgra and Shâmbavî, the person's gaze focuses on a single point, squinting (voluntary squinting) either at the middle of the forehead (Shâmbavî) or at the tip of the nose (Nasikâgra)[1]. Nasikâgra *mudrâ* is also used as a support in certain yoga meditations. The tip of the nose is also an energy center. While concentrating on the point, try to balance left and right vision.

Here, we will alternate successively (1) *Shâmbavî mudrâ*, gaze directed towards the middle of the forehead, (2) *Bhoochari mudrâ*, gaze into the void, without using the hands, (3) *Nasikâgra mudrâ*, gaze on the nose and (4) relaxation of the eyes, motionless. This forms a cycle.

Stay for about 10 seconds on each *mudrâ*, with your eyes open, and finish by relaxing your eyes, open or closed, which you can extend as long as your mind remains calm and focused.

Perform several cycles in this way, then concentrate for a few moments.

N° 42 – PREPARING FOR SHÂMBAVÎ MUDRÂ

If you have difficulty learning *Shâmbavî mudrâ*, you can also start with the following exercise:

△ Inhale slowly and adopt *Shâmbavî mudrâ*, eyes open, squinting towards the middle of the forehead.

▽ Exhale slowly and relax your eyes (eyes closed).

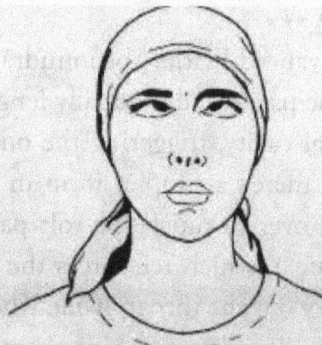

Shâmbavî mudrâ

---

1. Nasikâgra: literally the tip of the nose.

N° 43 – SAMATÂ PRÂNÂYÂMA AND NASIKÂGRA MUDRÂ ★★★

Nasikâgra mudrâ

△ Inhale slowly, evenly, with your gaze and concentration on the tip of your nose.

▽ Exhale with the same concentration.

Practice for a dozen breaths.

Breathe long and evenly and be receptive to the vibration. This exercise brings out the vibration of prâna.

Then prolong concentration on Mûlâdhâra or on the heart without worrying about breathing.

If concentration wanes, repeat the whole exercise.

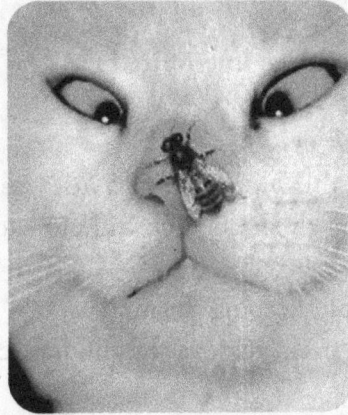

Nasikâgra mudrâ cat version

N° 44 – KAKI MUDRÂ ★★★

Inhalation and exhalation are accompanied by the Nasikâgra mudrâ, with the gaze directed towards the tip of the nose.

△ The inspiration here is taken through the mouth. The lips tighten in a circle to form the sound O. This position of the mouth is called Kaki mudrâ, the gesture of the crow. Concentrate as if you were drinking prâna.

▽ Exhale slowly and evenly through the nose. Maintain concentration on the prâna.

Kaki mudrâ is an exceptional practice for feeling and connecting with prâna.

The following two mudras are practices related to meditation.

N° 45 – ÛRDHVA MUKHA PRÂNÂYÂMA ★★★

In square breathing, Samavrittî prânâyâma, for example, 6 : 6 : 6 : 6.

△ Inhale as you lift your chin to the maximum and take the *Shâmbavî mudrâ* + *Mûla bandha*.

▲ Hold the breath for 6 seconds, keeping *Shâmbavî* and *Mûla bandha*.

▽ Exhale in 6 seconds, while bringing the head back and relaxing the eyes, but keep *Mûla bandha*.

▼ Remove Mûla bandha and relax in vacuum retention for 6 seconds.

Practice three breaths. Then close and relax your eyes and body. With practice, you'll be able to increase the rhythm and link more cycles together.

This prânâyâma leads to deep interiorization.

N° 46 – ÂKÂSHI MUDRÂ ★★★

△ Inhale in Ujjâyî, with *Khecarî and Shâmbavî mudrâs* while stretching the neck and tilting the head back without excess. Leave the glottis semi-open.

Breathe in this position, keeping the mudras.

Then bring the head back, remove the mudras, close the eyes and remain inward.

Practice several breaths according to your ability, then relax and awaken your receptivity.

Proceed with caution. If you feel dizzy, strongly contract the *Mûla bandha*. If you cannot avoid dizziness, abandon this practice.

Mudras and dynamizing bandhas

N° 47 – THE PRACTICE OF MÛLA BANDHA ★★★

Mûla bandha, the contraction of the base (*Mûla*), consists in contracting, in an upward movement, the anus and perineum[1]. It can be made more effective by also contracting the abdominal muscles below the navel and placing a small cushion under the buttocks to create pressure on the perineum. In yoga, the anus and perineum are two distinct energy cen-

1. In the higher version of the practice, concentration on the perineum is replaced by concentration on the base chakra, Mûlâdhâra.

ters. Depending on the orientation of the practice, concentration may be on the perineum or on another energy center.[1]

The stronger the contraction, the greater the effectiveness of this bandha.[2]

Mûla bandha is a practice that structures, gathers, strengthens, gathers and raises *prâna* and the psyche to a higher vibratory level.

Its role is to control and increase internal energy. This *bandha* is indispensable for breath-holding with full lungs (*kumbhaka*), amplifying the effectiveness of prânâyâma and enhancing our energetic and psychic defences. It is therefore an excellent anti-emotional practice, linked to inner strength, stability and confidence. *Mûla bandha* is inseparable from energetic yoga practices, in which it is often spontaneously introduced.

N° 48 – THE PRACTICE OF ASHWINÎ MUDRÂ ★★★

Let's listen to what the Gueranda Samhita, one of the classic texts of Hatha Yoga, has to say about it:

Contract and dilate the anus passage again and again. This is called Ashwinî mudrâ. It facilitates the awakening of the Shakti (Kundalinî). This Ashwinî is a great mudrâ; it eliminates all diseases linked to the rectum. It brings strength and vigour and prevents premature death. – Guerand Samhitâ[3]

Ashwinî mudrâ, the mare mudrâ, involves alternately contracting and relaxing the sphincters of the anus.

We describe two methods: the first performs contraction and relaxation over several seconds, synchronized with breathing; the second performs contraction very rapidly, at a rate of around two seconds per contraction/relaxation. Note that some schools replace relaxation by dilation, with an outward thrust. In all cases, maximum contraction and relaxation are essential.

First (preliminary) method

Make yourself comfortable in a seated position. You can place a small layer under the perineum to make the exercise easier.

1. Above the perineum, in the subtle physique, lies the Kanda, the meeting place of all nâdîs.

2. There is a second, more internal sphincter. You need to be able to feel the contraction in the spine rising to the level of the diaphragm.

3. *Guerand Samhitâ* is a traditional Hatha Yoga scripture.

△ Inhale for 2-3 seconds while contracting the anus to the maximum. Simultaneous contraction of the buttocks is tolerated at first.

▽ Exhale in 2 or 3 seconds and relax the muscles of the anus, synchronizing with the exhale.

This constitutes a cycle. Practice 20 to 50 cycles progressively.

Second method

You may or may not synchronize rectal contractions/relaxations with breathing.

Suddenly and completely contract the sphincters of the anus, then immediately relax the anus completely. Make sure you relax completely after each contraction, if you want to make it last as long as possible. To do this, as in the first method, rely on the rhythm. Perform the contraction-relaxation in one second, but in two (one-two, one-two, one-two, one-two...).

Gradually perform 20 to 50 contractions/relaxations.

Superior practice

If you want to intensify the experience, you can experience the ascension of this fundamental force-consciousness, at the origin of all our evolution, without triggering the dazzling awakening of Kundalinî.

When you're comfortable with this practice, increase it by 10 contractions / relaxations a day until you reach 108. During contractions, concentrate on balancing the left/right energy body.

Then close your eyes and go inward to feel the movement of prâna in the pelvis. As you perfect your technique, you'll become capable of a much stronger contraction, and you'll gradually feel the prâna rise in Sushumnâ.

This constitutes a cycle.

Progressively perform 3 cycles of 108 and prolong the concentration that follows the exercise. You'll be able to experience the physical senses of internal energy in no time.

By increasing your own consciousness-strength in this way, you will increase the energy throughout your body/mind system and discover the force of individual evolution, the dynamic part of the Spiritual Force, which eliminates all depression, all weariness, and propels the individual into the flow of his or her destiny.

However, as human nature is so complex, don't insist on abandoning the practice if you quickly experience unpleasant physical symptoms, strong negative impressions and emotions or unusual psychic experiences during your apprenticeship. You can replace it with the practice of yoga postures and alternate breathing, Nâdî Shodana, with moderate retentions.

It's worth noting that Indian spiritual yoga[1] has traditionally been reserved for individuals of sound mind and body, and that many Indian masters considered, not without reason, that we Westerners often suffer from psychological problems. Today, with the generalization of consumer society, all human beings have psychological problems. This is vividly demonstrated today by the enthronement of so many presidents and heads of state – supposedly belonging to humanity's elite, yet individually egotistical, extremist, extravagant, depraved, unstable, neurotic and tyrannical. How long ago it was in ancient Indian civilizations that kings were sages and yogis, the guarantors of balance and order in the world[2]!

It's also worth noting that the growth of strength-consciousness at the heart of life is one of the developments of Sri Aurobindo's yoga.

N° 49 – PRACTISING VAJROLÎ MUDRÂ AND ACTIVATING THE NÂDÎ AROHAN ★★★

The chakra's location is threefold: central, frontal and posterior (dorsal). The central part feeds the chakra's deep, occult and fundamental existence; the frontal existence concerns the chakra's influence on the psyche and its external, everyday functioning. The posterior part of the chakra, located in the back and rear of the body, is linked to our past, our subconscious.

We've seen Ashwinî mudrâ and Mûla bandha. They activate the most important nâdî, Sushumnâ, at spinal level, which feeds the central part of the chakras.

But there's another way to feed the chakras – and that's through their

---

1. Note the distinction made by Indians between spiritual and cultural (or hygienic) yoga. Cultural or hygienic yoga has spread to the West, and more recently to India, with the spread of yoga in schools and posture competitions (âsanas).

2. You can still get an idea of this in some of our root peoples.

frontal area. The chakra in Sushumnâ is similar to the center of a vortex, and this vortex unfolds in front of the frontal surface of the body. And all chakras, in their frontal existence, are linked to a nâdî, complementary to Sushumnâ. In this context, Swami Satyananda Saraswati calls the central nâdî (Sushumnâ) "Awarohan" and the frontal nâdî "Arohan. They seem to correspond to the Chinese Governor and Conception vessels.

Just as Sushumnâ is activated by Mûla bandha and Ashwinî mudrâ, so Vajrolî mudrâ activates the "Arohan nâdi.

This is why the practice of Vajrolî mudrâ plays a complementary role, particularly important when we are concerned with our daily external life.

The practice

This practice mirrors Ashwinî mudrâ, but involves the front of the body. Contract suddenly and completely the muscles in the lower abdomen responsible for your urge to urinate, or rather its retention, i.e. at genital level.

Intensely contract this muscle (as if you were trying to stop the flow of urine). Then immediately relax it completely. Make sure you relax after each contraction. To do this, as in the first method, rely on the rhythm. Carry out the contraction-relaxation over two seconds, in two different beats (one-two, one-two, one-two, one-two...).

To isolate the muscles and differentiate them from those used for Mûla bandha and Ashwinî mudrâ, the position of the pelvis is different in both cases.

For Mûla and Ashwinî, place a cushion under the perineum and bring the pelvis forward to isolate the rectum area, but for Vajrolî mudrâ, on the contrary, arch the back as much as possible and concentrate on the lower frontal area of the abdomen, balancing the left and right parts.

Practice 20 to 50 contractions / relaxations progressively. You may or may not synchronize contractions / relaxations with breathing.

As we have seen, Vajrolî increases prâna in the frontal nâdî. It is therefore an excellent practice for prostate problems and probably also for regulating gynaecological symptoms. It's also an excellent health practice.

N° 50 – UDDÎYÂNA BANDHA ★★★

The word "Uddîyâna" means upward movement.

Uddîyâna bandha consists of exhaling fully, closing the glottis – i.e. with empty lungs – releasing the belly and expanding the ribcage, as if to inhale. This triggers a depression, a vacuum in the ribcage, which draws the diaphragm and organs upwards, pulling in the belly. To succeed, you need to relax your abdominal muscles.

It's usually learned standing, legs half-bent, hands resting on thighs, elbows outwards. This amplifies the movement.

But you can also do it lying on your back. The exercise is easier, but less intense.

Uddîyâna bandha should be performed on an empty stomach, and will be more successful if the bowels are emptied. This bandha is contra-indicated for people with heart problems, high blood pressure, gastric ulcers and, of course, pregnant women. It is excellent for stimulating all digestive functions and increasing general vitality. Uddîyâna bandha and all the variants described here are ideal to prepare for the practice of prânâyâma with retentions.

It is more difficult to perform in a seated position. The knees must be in contact with the floor. In this case, the best position is Padmâsana, the Lotus.

From a standing position, as described above, take a full, deep breath.

Exhale fully, keep your lungs empty and close your glottis, relax your abdominal muscles and expand your ribcage. Keep your belly tucked in as far as possible, pressing down on your hands for as long as you feel comfortable. You'll feel a depression in your throat, a sign that the practice has been well executed. Once you've mastered the technique, concentrate with your eyes closed on the prâna in the belly area during the practice.

Then release the belly and raise the head before breathing in again and relaxing. Use this moment of relaxation to focus on the perception of prâna in the body.

Practice 3 to 10 times.

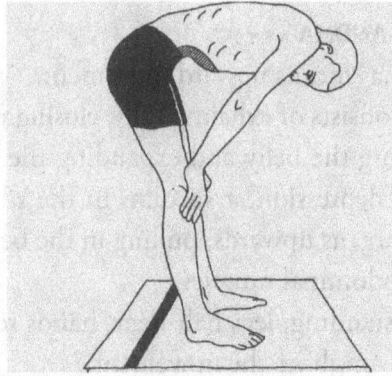

Uddîyâna bandha
In the above drawing, the legs are straight.
They can be bent halfway for greater stability

N° 51 – UDDÎYÂNA BANDHA CASCADE

Stand up, exhale fully, close the glottis and remain with empty lungs for the duration of the practice. Assume the Uddîyâna bandha position, and perform a rapid succession of **retractions** (*Uddîyâna*) and **relaxations** of the belly (on empty lungs), then push the belly forward, inhale gently and return to the normal standing position. Catch your breath and relax for a few moments, before repeating a few series if necessary.

In this variant, the effort is placed on each suction/retraction movement of the abdomen (the relaxation that follows each retraction is passive).

The concentration is the same, on the prâna.

N° 52 – AGNISÂRA DHAUTI ★★★

This practice – like all variants of Uddîyâna bandha – increases the digestive fire and brings great vitality.

Perform a rapid, alternating succession of abdominal **retractions** (*Uddîyâna*) and **expansions** (inflating the abdominal muscles). This is what distinguishes it from the previous exercise.

Equalize the duration of inward inhalation and outward expansion. This exercise is followed by concentration on prâna.

N° 53 – UDDÎYÂNA BANDHA + JÂLANDHARA BANDHA ★★★

Standing or sitting, perform the Uddîyâna bandha with the Jâlandhara bandha, compressing the neck with the chin.

N° 54 – UDDÎYÂNA BANDHA + MÛLA BANDHA ★★★

In a standing position, or lying down if you have not mastered the bandha in a seated position, perform Uddîyâna bandha to which you will add Mûla bandha, contracting the anus.

To return, release, in order: Mûla bandha, then the belly, then the glottis before breathing in again.

N° 55 – UDDÎYÂNA B + ASHWINÎ MUDRÂ ★★★

Here's a more powerful variant than the previous exercise. Take the Uddîyâna bandha position, retracting the abdomen, and for the duration of the empty retention, instead of the Mûla bandha, perform a series of contractions/relaxations of the anus in Ashwinî mudrâ,

N° 56 – TRIANGULAR PRÂNÂYÂMA (SHUNYAKA) + ½ UDDÎYÂNA BANDHA

Begin triangular breathing on empty lungs, equalizing the three beats.

Then add half an Uddîyâna, without forcing, with a slight withdrawal of the belly in the empty retention.

Afterwards, you can double the Shunyaka time. This will enable you to hold the bandha longer.

Once you've got the hang of it, you can add *Mûla bandha* and concentration on the base chakra, Mûlâdhâra.

▼ With shunyaka, rhythm **(1 : 1 : 2)** for example + ½ *Uddîyâna bandha* + *Mûla bandha* + Mûlâdhâra centering.

N° 57 – FROM UDDÎYÂNA BANDHA TO CENTRAL NAULI

Nauli is a superior exercise requiring good abdominal muscles and mastery of Uddiyâna bandha.

The easiest way is to learn it lying on your back, legs slightly bent, feet on the ground.

In the supine position, head on the floor, exhale fully, withdraw the abdomen into Uddîyâna bandha, remain with empty lungs, glottis closed, and raise the head and upper back slightly, taking care to maintain the bandha. This will trigger a contraction of the abdominal muscles, known as the rectus abdominis, producing an outgrowth of these muscles in the middle of the abdomen. Prolong this contraction, keeping the abdomen withdrawn for as long as possible. Then relax for a few moments before repeating several times.

When you've mastered it, practice standing, then sitting. Add the Mûla bandha.

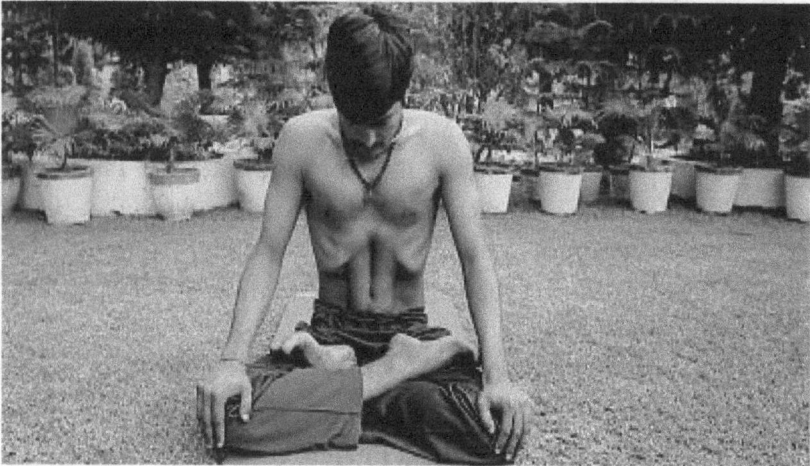

Central Nauli

N° 58 – TRIBANDHA + SHUNYAKA ★★★

Tribandha integrates the three bandhas: Uddîyâna, Jâlandhara and Mûla. It's a classic yet powerful exercise. It is generally performed in a seated position, but can also be done standing up.

△ Inhale deeply.

▽ Exhale deeply.

▲ Take the Jâlandhara bandha, flexing the head and remaining with empty lungs.

Then add Uddîyâna bandha and finally Mûla bandha. Hold the three bandhas for the duration of the vacuum retention.

When you want to return, proceed in reverse order: remove the Mûla bandha, then the Uddîyâna, then raise your head before inhaling.

Relax well before repeating 2 or 3 times.

Once you're used to it, you can add concentration while holding the three bandhas, either on Âjnâ chakra or on Mûlâdhâra.

Advanced âsana practitioners can practice it in demi-Pince. There are several variations.

This is a superior Hatha Yoga practice. It positively and strongly influences the endocrine system, stimulates the digestive system, strengthens the nervous system, stabilizes prâna and the psyche, and increases vitality and consciousness-strength, Shakti. Combined with concentration on the chakras during and after practice, it has the power of true meditation.

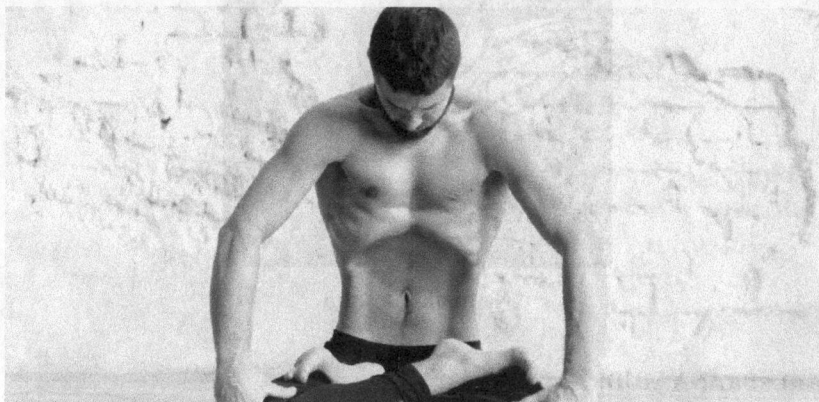

Tribandha

N° 59 – TRIBANDHA + CENTRAL NAULI ★★★

The practice is identical to the previous exercise. Nauli is added to Uddîyâna.

> *The practice of all these bandhas linked to the belly chakra, Manipura, is important for developing the perception and manipulation of prâna. This is achieved by concentrating on prâna during and after practice.*

N° 60 – SÛRYA PRÂNÂYÂMA MUDRÂ

This mudrâ is practiced over 9 days at sunrise.

Seated, hands clasped, in *Namaskâra mudrâ*, practice **Sâvitrî prânâyâma**, slower and slower, adding units each day. Start at **8 – 4 – 8 – 4** until **24 – 12 – 24 – 12**.

△ Inhale: raise your hands, still clasped, open them and turn your palms towards the sun, keeping your thumbs and forefingers together to create an opening through which you can look at the sun.

▲ Kumbhaka: receptivity to sun prâna.

▽ Exhale: bring the hands back to the chest in Namaskâr mudrâ.

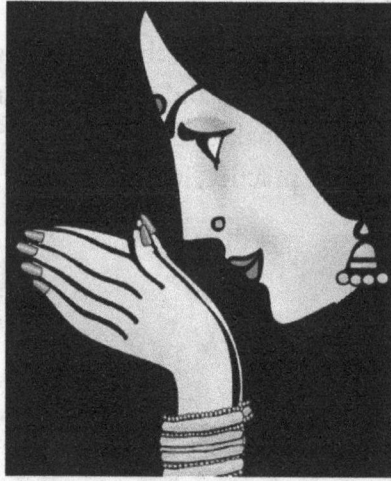

Namaskâr mudrâ

N° 61 – PRÂNA MUDRÂ

In a seated meditation position, hands on thighs, exhale and hold the breath for a few seconds with *Mûla bandha* and concentration in Mûlâdhâra.

△ As you inhale, move your hands upwards, palms facing the body, close to the abdomen, towards the head, concentrating simultaneously on the prâna rising in Sushumnâ[1], from Mûlâdhâra to Sahasrâra.

▲ In kumbhaka, the hands are raised and spread out above the head with a double concentration: on Sahasrâra and on universal Prâna, or on sending vibrations of peace to all beings.

▽ Exhaling, the hands return to the thighs and the prâna descends towards Mûlâdhâra.

1. Sushumnâ is the central subtle channel (nâdî) in the spinal column.

Prânâyâma:
The Path to Meditation

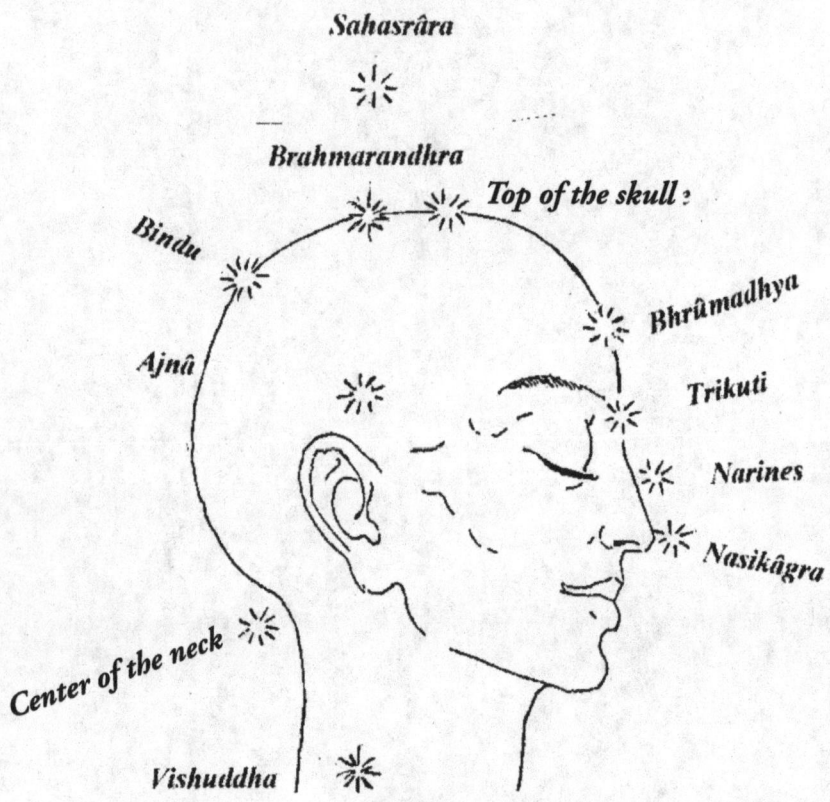

Sahasrâra

Brahmarandhra

Top of the skull ?

Bindu

Bhrûmadhya

Ajnâ

Trikuti

Narines

Nasikâgra

Center of the neck

Vishuddha

Head energy centers

XI
INTRODUCTION
TO SUBTLETIES

The synergy of breath and concentration

By combining certain concentrations with breathing, we can amplify the benefits of both, and we can orient exercises differently to give them new properties.

On the other hand, the regular practice of prânâyâma does not necessarily imply the manipulation and use of prâna. To manipulate prâna, we need to perceive it. Subtle breathing leads us there.

The vibratory subtlety of prâna

N° 62 – BREATHING PERFUME ★★★

Focus your attention and sensitivity on the nostrils, inhaling as you would the scent of a flower. The delicate sensations are then localized at the top of the nostrils, towards the olfactory zone. At this point, you can observe that the breath slows down and a subtle vibration appears, which can be reproduced on the exhale with the same concentration. If you close your eyes, a luminosity may even appear at the base of the forehead, in *Trikutî*, and a state of relaxation enters the mind.

This is an important exercise. It opens the door to all the subtlety in the breath, and is therefore a necessary foundation.

N° 63 – SENSATIONS IN THE NOSTRILS ★★★

In this exercise, we focus our attention on the sensations caused by the passage of the breath through the nostrils: sensations of warmth as we exhale, sensations that move towards the top of the nose, towards the forehead, as we inhale, and that descend as we exhale. Then concentrate successively on the three zones inside the nostrils: the lower, middle and upper parts, taking ten breaths or so for each zone, and concentrating on the entire inner perimeter of the nostrils.

Finally, complete the exercise by accompanying the movement of sensations up and down the inner walls, synchronizing this movement with your breathing. Pay equal attention to each nostril. The lower part relates to the body; the middle part to the vital and emotional being; the upper part to the mind. We know that there are nerve endings in the nose that are connected to the various organs of the body. This is why this exercise can be considered complete, and why its influence extends to the whole human being.

N° 64 – EXPANDING NOSTRILS

After practicing the previous exercise, concentrating on the passage of the breath through the nostrils, from bottom to top on the inhale, and from top to bottom on the exhale, between the base of the nostrils and Trikutî, you can continue with this higher variant, which requires great subtlety in the search for sensations.

Imagine that at the precise point where the breath passes through, the passage dilates and widens.

It's easier to succeed in this exercise by concentrating more on the subtle nostrils, in our etheric double[1], than on the physical ones. If you succeed, relaxation can lead to sweetness, bliss and a feeling of inner light.

N° 65 – SAMATÂ PRÂNÂYÂMA ★★★

Samatâ[2] prânâyâma is a subtle breath in which inhalation and exhalation are equalized in duration and the breath is made regular and uniform, like the flow of a trickle of oil or the movement of a great still river. But what makes it so effective is the slowness with which it is performed. In so doing, the VIBRATION of prâna emerges, plunging mind and

---

1. Yoga, like all ancient traditions, associates with the physical world a subtle, de-localized layer, inaccessible to our gross senses. The terms *pranic, etheric* or *subtle physical* are synonymous.

2. Samatâ: equality of soul, balance.

body into a gentle, harmonious bliss. The hallmark of this prânâyâma is the presence of prânic vibration.

The training we have undergone in lengthening inhalation and exhalation prepares us here for the discovery of the subtlety of prâna vibration and the equanimity so necessary for meditation.

N° 66 – SAMATÂ PRÂNÂYÂMA AND BREATH SUSPENSION

In deep relaxation, focus your attention on your breathing, equalizing the duration of the inhalation and exhalation. Gradually, your breath will slow down. At this point, enter into the subtlety of the breath by lengthening it as much as possible, then become aware of its suspension between inhalation and exhalation (kumbhaka) and between exhalation and inhalation (shunyaka). This is the most important part of the exercise, so don't miss it.

(N° 43) – NASIKÂGRA MUDRÂ + SAMATÂ PRÂNÂYÂMA ★★★

Practice Samatâ prânâyâma while concentrating on the tip of your nose. Concentrate on perceiving the vibration of prâna.

N° 67 – AUM AND BREATHING ★★★

This exercise is performed in three stages, which complement and reinforce each other. Don't be tempted to perform only the last one.

Place your attention in the nostrils and equalize inhalation and exhalation until you obtain a naturally long, even breath. At this point, add the sound AUM. Sing it inwardly several times on the inhale and several times on the exhale. The final nasal sound should be as long as the vowels.

Next, vibrate the *prânava*[1] once during the entire inhalation and once during the exhalation.

In the third stage, the sound of the mantra extends over the entire duration of a breath, with the vowels on the inhale and the nasal sound on the exhale. The slower AUM is chanted, the more powerful its effect. Each step must last long enough for the breath and sound to merge.

For Easterners, this sound represents the sound of Universal Consciousness, or the fundamental vibration of the universe. But you don't need

---

1. The *prânava* refers to the AUM mantra.

to believe in Eastern philosophies to benefit from it, nor will its practice make you a Hindu or Buddhist. So don't hesitate to sing it and discover its beauty, its power to relax, expand and internalize. This sound is unique, it belongs to humanity as a whole, and is not interchangeable with any other sound in any other language. It represents what unites man with his deepest nature, what unites man with man, and what unites man with all creation. It is the sound of unity.

N° 68 – SAMATÂ PRÂNÂYÂMA AND AUM ★★★

Place your attention in the nostrils and equalize inhalation and exhalation until you obtain a naturally long, even breath. At this point, add the sound AUM. Vibrate the *prânava* once during the entire inhalation and once during the exhalation. The final nasal sound should be as long as the vowels.

The slower AUM is sung, the deeper and more powerful its effect. If perception of the vibration in Samatâ prânâyâma is difficult, the contribution of AUM makes it accessible to all.

N° 69 – KRIYÂ: OVERALL RELAXATION WITH AUM ★★★

△ Inhale and bring the subtle breath up to the *Trikutî* point.
▲ Hold your breath for a few seconds in Trikutî.
▽ Exhale slowly, pushing the Trikutî prâna towards Bhrûmadhya, in the middle of the forehead, and enter the cranium to relax the whole brain. Take about ten breaths.

Then continue with the complete exercise:

△▲ Proceed in the same way for inspiration and retention, up to Trikuti.
▽ As you exhale, while mentally associating the sound AUM, spread the relaxation vibration from Trikutî to Bhrûmadhya, then to the brain, then to the cerebellum and finally to the entire spinal cord.

Proceed in stages if necessary. Take about ten breaths.

This exercise is called a *Kriyâ*[1].

N° 70 – SHEETALI AND SÎTKÂRI, SUMMER PRÂNÂYÂMAS ★★★

Summer prânâyâmas are effective for cooling the body, but above all,

---

1. *Kriyâ Yoga*, see chapter 17.

they are prâna pumps. The slower the breath, the more effective they are. There are several other variations.

Summer prânâyâmas are characterized by inhalation through the mouth and exhalation through the nose.

Variant 1: Sîtkâri prânâyâma

△ In Sîtkâri, the practitioner makes the SSS sound. To do this, the lips are parted as in smiling, and the inhalation is made through clenched teeth, with the tongue against the teeth.

Variant 2: Sheetali prânâyâma

In Sheetali, the tongue sticks out, and the lips tighten the outer edges, as if to form the sound O. This curls the tongue around itself, forming a tube through which inspiration takes place.

▽ Exhalation takes place through the nose.

Inhale the prâna through the mouth and maintain concentration on the prâna as you exhale.

You'll amplify the effects by concentrating on prâna in short, full-lunged retention.

N° 71 – THE BREATHING OF THE BEE, BHRÂMARÎ, THE MODERATE FORM
★★★

In this prânâyâma, the nasal sound MMM is emitted on exhaling, with the mouth closed and the ears plugged with the fingers.

Adopt a correct sitting position, balanced with your back straight. Close your eyes and mouth, inhale deeply, cover your ears and pronounce the nasal sound aloud, exhaling as slowly and evenly as possible. Then hold the breath for a few seconds on empty lungs.

While exhaling and in *shunyaka,* concentrate on the inner sounds or the memory of the sound AUM. This constitutes a cycle.

Aim for maximum resonance by opening the jaws, which should be loose, and exerting more or less pressure on the ear. You should reach a very high resonance in which, with a little practice, you'll be able to distinguish several sounds, including at least one low-pitched and one high-pitched one. This is the creation of *harmonics.*

Practice a minimum of five to ten cycles, gradually; you can breathe normally between cycles if you're a little out of breath, but keep listening, keeping your ears plugged. At the end of the chant, continue to listen to the inner sounds that often appear at this point.

This very pleasant prânâyâma is particularly effective in relieving mental tension, dissolving negative emotions, eliminating energy blockages and inducing interiorization. On a physical level, it can reduce certain types of high blood pressure and improve the voice. It is a practice of the yoga of sounds, Nâda yoga.

Concentrate on the sounds with great subtlety and at the same time on the inner state of relaxation and well-being, which can go as far as inner bliss when training is advanced.

We now turn to a more advanced form of prânâyâma, in which a sound is also emitted on inspiration.

N° 72 – THE COMPLETE BEE'S BREATH: THE SOUND OF BREATHING IN AND OUT ★★★

The inspiratory and expiratory sounds, which are different, are said to correspond to the female and male bees. In any case, the inspiratory sound is very high-pitched. You can learn it by singing aloud **during inspiration** a sound somewhere between the Hiiiii and the Huuu. Practice in the same way, striving for a regular, even sound.

Once you've mastered it, practice Bhrâmarî prânâyâma with the low, nasal sound on the exhale and the high sound on the inhale.

After a moment, which you feel is sufficient, stop the prânâyâma and listen to the inner sound.

VARIANT – THE BEE + CONCENTRATION ★★★

Raise the high-pitched sound of the inhale to the upper parts of the head or above, and bring the lower-pitched sound of the exhale to the pelvis, or more precisely to the base chakra, Mûlâdhâra, if you can find it. We'll see later.

The vibratory subtlety of consciousness

N° 73 – THE PSYCHIC FILTER

There's a lot of talk these days about pollution and air quality. Yoga adds a psychic atmosphere, made up of all the mental, emotional and other emanations of the people who live there. This psychic atmosphere is obviously not the same in a forest or in a city, where millions of little vibrations of egoism, greed, fear or restlessness mix together, forming an aura that is characteristic of cities.

The practice of yoga also teaches us that thought is a realizing force, whether constructive or destructive, and uses it in many techniques.

△ Breathe in the white light, the spiritual light that generates psychic purification.

▽ Exhale as you visualize the color black, rejecting all negative thoughts and dark movements of consciousness. You can also breathe out a particular defect you wish to detach yourself from.

N° 74 – COLORED BREATHING

Begin to focus on your breathing, gradually lengthening your breath. When your breath is calm and full, associate it with the color. Inhale the seven colors in the same order: one breath for each of red, orange and yellow; then three breaths for green; then five breaths for blue, indigo and violet.

You can bring this color into the head if you're looking for mental energization, or into the lungs, into the whole body, or more specifically into a weak or diseased organ.

Continue your practice until you feel a concrete sense of strength, self-confidence or healing.

Breathe in the energy and atmosphere of the color for a long time.

VARIATION – THE RAINBOW PRÂNÂYÂMA, TRIANGULAR PRÂNÂYÂMA IN KUMBHAKA

In this triangular prânâyâma with kumbhaka, visualize the 7 colors of the rainbow in turn (one or more breaths per color) and end with the whole rainbow.

△ Inhale the color.

▲ Concentrate on the color.

▽ Spread the colored energy throughout your body.

N° 75 – THE PERFECT CURVE ★★★

This breathing consists of three stages, each as important as the others. It is here, at this moment, through your breath, in the Samatâ prânâyâma, that you can experience the present. Don't look for any usefulness or purpose in this exercise. It's there to guide you, to carry you away, to transport you into the present moment.

The first phase consists of slowing down your breathing and stabilizing your attention on the inhale and exhale.

In the second phase, you will focus your attention on the subtle perception of breath suspensions after the inhale and after the exhale. Note that these are suspensions, not retentions. Breathing should remain natural, albeit slow and even.

Finally, in the third phase, the suspensions will take the form of a curve between the two movements of the breath. Enter into the mystery of this passage from one state to another, this change between two antagonistic and complementary states symbolized by this curve.

End with a short meditation on silence.

N° 76 – MOVEMENT IN STILLNESS ★★★

This breathing requires great availability and subtlety.

Start by equalizing inhalation and exhalation and regulating the flow of breath with a uniform sound and flow (Samatâ prânâyâma).

When you've internalized, at the end of the inhalation, during the breath suspension, continue the inhalation in imagination, and at the end of the exhalation, during the empty suspension, prolong the exhalation in the same way.

N° 77 – INSPIRATION IN EXHALATION AND EXHALATION IN INSPIRATION ★★★

Through Samatâ prânâyâma, introduce subtlety into your thinking.

Next, gather your awareness to achieve a double concentration in which you imagine you're breathing out as you inhale, and you imagine you're breathing in as you exhale.

XII
PRÂNÂYÂMA:
BREATH RETENTION

Male and female prâna

Prâna is the energy of life. The principle of life is achieved through energy, power and enjoyment. Power is active, masculine; enjoyment is passive, feminine. In relation to meditation, it's useful to distinguish two forms of prâna, which we'll call: masculine prâna and feminine prâna.

Male prâna

Masculine prâna is related to Kumbhaka, the retention of breath with full lungs. It vibrates with strength and energy. It is linked to nâdî Pingalâ, the right side of the body, and to Sushumnâ, the central channel. It is linked to stability of citta and psyche, balance, vigilance, equality of soul, inner strength and power, vitality, energy, expansion, self-confidence, concentration, dynamism, motivation, enterprise, authority, taking charge and achieving goals. It creates an individualized, mature, responsible and autonomous human being. It is a considerable resource for external life, as much for intellectual and vital life as for action. It increases consciousness-strength. However, this can lead to ego-strengthening and must therefore be controlled by the inner being, the Psychic Being, the Soul. We can see here that the development of feminine prâna is highly recommended to balance the personality.

In meditation, if the disciple is well guided, masculine prâna leads to the awakening of Kundalinî and to Raja Yoga meditation in an increasingly deep and unified concentration. Here too, the cultivation of feminine prâna is a necessity.

Technically speaking, in addition to kumbhaka, practices that develop male prâna include strength and backbending postures, Uddîyâna bandha and all its variants, Nauli, Ashwinî mudrâ and Mûla bandha.

Female prâna

Feminine prâna is linked to empty retention, shunyaka. It is the uniform, uninterrupted, subtle, peaceful and balancing vibration that brings harmony and bliss, and takes us deep within, towards the deep heart and unity of all beings. It vibrates with the prânava AUM. It is poetry and music that carries harmony.

It leads to peace, balance and interiorization, and raises vibratory quality. Feminine prâna brings sensitivity and receptivity to the sensory and emotional spheres, leading to stability of the citta in gentleness, peace and harmony. It draws us into inner bliss and wholeness, away from the ceaseless motion of outer life and nature. It is linked to nâdî Ida, the left side of the body, and to Sushumnâ, the central channel.

The practices that develop it are the balancing and polarizing postures, the forward bending and stretching postures, the Lotus posture and the inverted poses. This is shunyaka without Uddîyâna bandha. These are the subtle breaths and Dynamic Dualities of chapter 17. These are most of the kriyâs, such as those described below. It is the combination of prâna and vibration not produced by contact between two objects. This sound is called *Anâhata* in India, and is natural in the space of the deep heart.

This vibration dissolves aggression; it opens, enlarges, dilates, extends, welcomes, understands, melts resistance, brings receptivity, connects all things. It brings dedication and devotion.

In meditation, feminine prâna leads to the opening of the heart, the pacification of negative emotions, the amplification of sensitivity, the elevation and subtlety of consciousness, and the increasingly tranquil, uniform interiorization towards deep identification.

Feminine prâna awakens all forms of enjoyment, from sensory pleasure to joy, and from joy to bliss. It's a great healing force and, naturally, a great resource.

Prâna meditation

We've seen the five centers used for meditation: *Sahasrâra*, the Thousand-Petaled Lotus, above the head; *Âjnâ*, in the head; *Anâhata*, the Heart chakra; *Mûlâdhâra*, the Base chakra; and *Sushumnâ*, the subtle central channel.

However, as we describe throughout this book, it is possible to achieve meditation through prâna. In particular, through subtle breathing and kriyâs. This opens and stimulates the Manipûra chakra in the solar plexus and connects us to universal prâna.

After a certain amount of practice, concentration on this chakra, like the five centers mentioned above, often leads us back to the Deep Heart and the presence of the Psychic Being.[1]

The Upanishads consider Prâna to be the radiant energy of the Universal Spiritual Force. It says[2] :

He discovered that prâna is Brahman.

The classical discipline of prânâyâma, the method

In its traditional form, prânâyâma in India incorporates **kumbhaka**[3], the retention of breath with full lungs.

The method includes mastery of abdominal breathing, followed by full breathing.

Then, if you intend to undertake the discipline of self-transformation through prânâyâma, which necessarily includes the use of breath-holding, you'll need to practise purifying breaths, such as bellows, and rebalancing breaths, particularly left/right, for several months.

From a technical point of view, mastery of the *Jâlandhara* and *Mûla* bandhas is essential for breath retention, particularly Kumbhaka, lasting more than ten seconds. Empty retention, without the *Uddîyâna bandha*, does not present the same difficulties. We also need to ensure that you learn all the gestures that enable you to practice and perfect prânâyâma without any mental tension, without any stress on the nervous and respi-

1. Of course, this experience only comes about if we integrate the individual Divine into our spiritual representation and purpose.

2. Taittirîya Upanishad.

3. In ancient texts, the word kumbhaka is synonymous with prânâyâma.

ratory systems, and without any energy imbalance.

We'll know if we're on the right track when prânâyâma brings us the characteristic sensations of mental calm, emotional stability, energetic balance, lightness of body and improved health, as well as a multitude of sensations of well-being, rapture and bliss, particularly in the representation of feminine prâna with kriyâs and Dynamic Dualities (chapter 17).

Our legitimate aim, if we take this discipline seriously, will be to acquire with practice a vibratory stability, an exceptional inner balance and strength, and an abundance of vitality that can serve as the basis for a fulfilled life despite the pitfalls of our crazy times, and that will help us access the depths of meditation.

Preparing for kumbhaka

Nº 78 – NETÎ KRIYÂ, the nasal shower ★★★

Netî kriyâ, the nasal shower, is one of the purification kriyâs of yoga. It is indispensable for the practice of prânâyâma.

This involves inserting the mouth of the pot (called *lota*) into one nostril and letting the water – slightly warm and salty – flow out through the other nostril. Half the pot for the left nostril, half for the right.

To prevent water from entering the throat, lean forward sufficiently and turn your head. Breathe through an open mouth and relax your face.

Then, traditionally, you blow hard through your nostrils to expel the rest of the water. But you can also simply use a handkerchief.

You can buy lota on the Internet. Otherwise, some teapots may be suitable.

Always use spring or mineral water. Avoid tap water. Do not use a solution that is too saline. The correct proportion is that of physiological serum and does not give any unpleasant sensation. If you use pure, salt-free water, you'll damage your sinuses. Try using a small spoonful of salt at first. Use whole, natural fine salt.

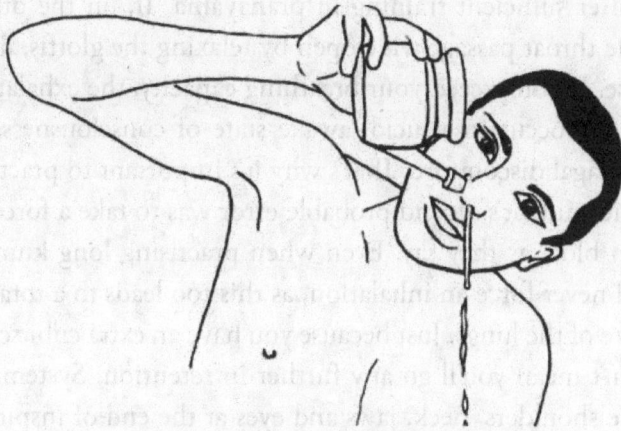

Jala netî, the nasal shower

A complementary variant of nasal cleansing, called **Sutra netî**, is performed by inserting a soft rubber probe inside the nostril and mouth. This is sometimes essential to clear the passage through the nostrils. Your yoga teacher can teach you how.

All this has a very positive effect on sinus health.

N° 79 – GLOTTIS CONTROL IN BREATH-HOLDING

Breath-holding with full lungs, when uncontrolled, can lead to dizziness or even fainting. This is a particular concern for freedivers, as an unconscious diver can breathe in water and drown.

The practice of prânâyâma with breath-holding—as well as the practice of yoga postures in kumbhaka[1]—accustoms the practitioner to anticipating its appearance, and to guard against it or stop it if it occurs.

To stop the discomfort instantly, you need to acquire the reflex of exhaling sharply through the mouth, as in exercise no. 19. But even then, the student must recognize that he has gone too far, and even if he has been able to escape the harmful consequences, he will need to learn the lesson for future practice.

However, this could have been avoided if he had cultivated glottis control. For when we close the glottis while holding our lungs full, we increase the pressure on the respiratory system. And this should only be

1. There is a method of practicing âsanas, popularized in the West by Sri Mahesh, in which full and empty suspensions are combined.

practised after sufficient training in prânâyâma. If, on the other hand, we leave the throat passage wide open by relaxing the glottis, discomfort cannot arise. If you exceed your breathing capacity, the exhalation reflex will inevitably occur in a lucid, awake state of consciousness, and will not trigger vagal discomfort. That's why it's important to practice glottis control. The student's second probable error was to take a forced breath, inhaling en bloc, as they say. Even when practising long kumbhaka(s), you should never force an inhalation, as this too leads to a totally useless overpressure of the lungs. Just because you have an extra cubic centimetre of air doesn't mean you'll go any further in retention. Systematic relaxation of the shoulders, neck, jaws and eyes at the end of inspiration will reinforce this habit.

The first exercise is to become aware of the swallowing reflex, as swallowing saliva closes the larynx by contracting (tightening) the glottis.

The second step is to learn to close the glottis voluntarily.

Take a moderate inspiration, without forcing, with the head straight, in balance, close the glottis for a few seconds and exhale gently after having unblocked the glottis. To unblock the glottis, breathe in again. Practice in this way until you've mastered the technique.

Then perform the same exercise, breathing in deeply but not excessively, as we've explained. This is essential training for learning prânâyâma.

The practice of Ujjâyî breathing is also excellent training for glottis control, as you learn to close the glottis to different degrees. In kumbhaka, the glottis is closed, but without pressure.

N° 80 – JÂLANDHARA BANDHA ★★★

Jâlandhara bandha consists of stretching the nape of the neck, then bending the head forward until the chin touches the hollow of the throat. If you've mastered Sarvângâsana, the Candle Posture, you'll easily master the technical aspect of Jâlandhara bandha.

During Kumbhaka, this bandha helps to contain prâna in the chest and ensure that it does not rise to the head, which would instantly trigger vertigo.

Vertigo is always an indication of a technical fault with harmful consequences.

There's another method in which the hands are placed on the thighs and the arms are extended, with the shoulders raised. This allows greater pressure of the chin against the throat. It is useful in the Tribandha (N° 58).

Performing Jâlandhara bandha in full- or empty-lung retention balances blood pressure and heartbeat, stimulates the thyroid and calms the mind. An excellent practice against stress, anxiety and anger.

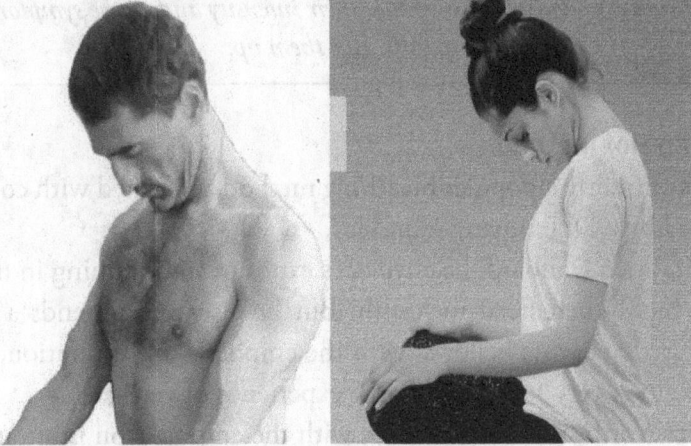

**The right position for breath retention
with the Jâlandhara bandha**

In breath retention, especially with full lungs (kumbhaka), the Jâlandhara bandha is associated with the Mûla bandha. Their function is to contain prâna inside the body and prevent it from escaping upwards and downwards. In so doing, they amplify internal pressure and the effectiveness of prânâyâma.

We'll practice the Jâlandhara bandha in the kumbhakas using the simple method. After preparing for the practice, with your back straight, shoulders relaxed and chest wide open, inhale deeply in full breath, with shoulders relaxed, stretch the neck and perform the Jâlandhara bandha, also blocking prâna with psychic closure. Use your will and imagination to seal the passage from top to bottom. Hold the prâna tightly with your mind, but keep your face, eyes and mind relaxed at all times. When you decide to exhale, raise your head, inhale a little air to unblock the glottis, then exhale slowly.

Do not breathe while holding the Jâlandhara bandha.

This bandha is not recommended for people with high blood pressure or heart problems. It can, however, be beneficial for thyroid problems. To balance blood pressure, the disorder must be slight and performed without the kumbhaka.

> *Training in your yogic disciplines should be carried out in such a way that unpleasant symptoms never occur during or after practice. If they do, modify them, reduce their intensity and, if the symptoms persist, give them up.*

The Wim Hof method

There's currently a popular breathing method associated with cold yoga, proposed by a Dutchman, Wim Hof.

Like Maurice Daubard, he advocates exposure and training in the cold. This is highly beneficial to health. But he also recommends a type of breathing that favors bellows, with the emphasis on inspiration, and he seems to look very favorably on the experience of vertigo.

In other words, two major errors, with the emphasis on inspiratory hyperventilation and the favoring of vertigo.

We can only deplore the improvised, inconsistent, dangerous and irresponsible teaching of such errors in relation to the age-old art of prânâyâma.

N° 81 – THE PRACTICE OF MÛLA BANDHA ★★★

Mûla bandha, the contraction of the base (*Mûla*), consists in contracting, in an upward movement, the anus and perineum[1]. It can be made more effective by also contracting the abdominal muscles below the navel and placing a small cushion under the buttocks to create pressure on the perineum. As kumbhaka progresses, abdominal contraction and Mûla bandha should also be strengthened. The best way to strengthen the muscles involved in the Mûla bandha is to practice Ashwinî mudrâ (see N° 48).

---

1. In the higher version of the practice, concentration on the perineum is replaced by concentration on the base chakra, Mûlâdhâra.

Physical preparation

The practice of prânâyâma with long breath-holding is inconceivable in India without assiduous practice of the postures, the âsanas. And ideally, âsanas precede prânâyâma.

However, we believe that a moderate practice of postures is sufficient to practice a moderate prânâyâma. In this case, breathing exercises and prânâyâmas will not involve long retentions, and will therefore not exceed about twenty seconds. On the other hand, the practice of alternate breathing will be particularly encouraged, and will be confined to the first three stages (see chapter 12).

Then, if you wish, you can deepen your prânâyâma practice.

On the other hand, before beginning prânâyâma with breath-holding, it's a good idea to relax the neck and do a few exercises to soften the legs and spine and free the breathing zones. Uddîyâna bandha and its variants are ideal before kumbhakas.

Ladies, during the first few days of your period, don't practice breath-holding and confine yourself to very moderate physical exercise. On the other hand, all practices related to feminine prâna are very favorable.

We'll assume you've assimilated the passage: *Learn to count without counting*, at the end of chapter 8.

N° 82 – KUMBHAKA: AN EXPERIENCE

Inhale deeply, then hold your breath with full lungs in kumbhaka. When the need to breathe arises, resist and keep your glottis closed. After a few seconds, you'll notice involuntary movements of the diaphragm and jerks in the abdominal muscles.

Experiment by remaining mentally relaxed, then unblock the glottis by breathing in again, before exhaling. Keep the mind relaxed during the experiment.

The prânâyâma session

A complete and balanced prânâyâma session can be divided into five parts:

1 – physical preparation

Physical preparation may include postures, a warm-up of the spine and legs, eye, neck and shoulder flexibility, and a short practice of Ashwinî mudrâ to tone the pelvic floor. B.K.S. Iyengar proposes an excellent exercise in a relaxed position, lying on the back with a thick cushion around the shoulder blades, to open the chest.

2 – releasing prâna
Bellows: Kapâlabhâti and Bhastrikâ, with variations as required. For example, 10 to 15 minutes.

3 – the concentration of prâna
Prânâyâma with breath-holding, Kumbhaka or shunyaka. For example, 20 to 30 minutes.

4 – the subtlety of prâna
Concentration prânâyâmas, such as variants with Ujjâyî, Samatâ prânâyâma, subtle breathing, Dynamic Dualities or kriyâs. For example, 15 minutes or more.

5 – static internalization
We'll finish with a more or less lengthy internalization, depending on our ability and availability.

However, there's no reason why you can't stop the session after the third part, and follow it with the same concentration (adopted during the retentions) maintained in deep internalization. You can also continue with kriyâs.

And of course, there's nothing to stop us sticking to the second part, followed by a meditation.

The transcendence of our vitality
N° 83 – PRÂNÂYÂMA WITH KUMBHAKA ★★★
Ideally, this breathing should always be practised in Nâdî Shodana, alternating breathing. Only if you have difficulty breathing through one nostril[1], should you choose normal breathing, inhaling through both

1. To unblock a nostril that is permanently or regularly obstructed, you need to perform a daily nasal wash, NETÎ (N° 96) with salt water and with the cord (catheter), SUTRA NETÎ. If the nasal septum is deformed, either at birth or by accident, the

nostrils together.

△ Inhale completely, **keeping your shoulders relaxed**. Do not inflate the belly completely. Open the ribcage as much as possible and raise the collarbones. Do not raise or contract your shoulders. When the breath reaches the top, don't try to breathe in more. It's always possible to gain a few cubic centimetres, but this would be at the cost of unnecessary and damaging tension.

Forced inspiration in kumbhakas leads to heart problems.

▲ Close the glottis. Perform *Jâlandhara bandha*, stretching the neck, raising the collarbones and lowering the chin against the throat. Hold the breath and perform *Mûla bandha*, the contraction of the base, with relaxed face and mind.

▽ Then remove *Mûla bandha*, remove *Jâlandhara bandha* by raising the head, clear the glottis by breathing in a little and exhale gently, letting the clavicles and ribcage descend slowly, finally contracting the abdominal strap to expel the air completely.

▼ Hold the breath for one or two seconds, then move on to the next breath.

Prânâyâma is practised with the eyes closed. The secret of successful breath-holding lies in muscular and, above all, mental relaxation, and inflexible concentration. In addition, sensory perception of prâna instantly facilitates kumbhaka.

The rhythms of kumbhaka
The basic rhythms of prânâyâma with Kumbhaka are:
1 : 2
1 : 1 :
1 : 2 : 2 ; (4 : 8 : 8)
1 : 3 : 2 ; (4 : 12 : 8)
1 : 4 : 2 ; (4 : 16 : 8)

operation may prove useful.

Nâdî Shodana, alternate breathing

1st stage: equalize inspiration and exhalation

2nd stage: double the exhalation (1:2); for example 4:8

3rd stage: introduction of the kumbhaka (1:1:2); for example 4:4:8

4st stage: rhythm (1 : 2 : 2); for example 4 : 8 : 8

5st stage: rhythm (1 : 4 : 2); for example 4 : 16 : 8

6th stage: rhythm (1 : 4 : 2 : 1) for example 4 : 16 : 8 : 4 and 5 : 20 : 10
: 5. After this rhythm comes :

7st stage: rhythm (1 : 6 : 4 : 2) e.g. 4 : 24 : 16 : 8 or 5 : 30 : 20 : 5.

> *Our first objective will be to achieve the classic rhythm: 4:16:8
> or better 5:20:10.*

We can then add concentration during retention. In all cases, develop your powers of observation and your sensitivity to prâna and inner atmospheres.

Then, if we're completely comfortable, we can go up to 4:16:8:4 or 5:20:10:5, while continuing to concentrate.

The characteristics of prâna

◊ Energy

The experience of prâna itself brings together five characteristics: *vibration and light, life, energy and balance*. Focusing on the energetic aspect will bring us the vibratory or psychological experience of life, energy and an unusual dynamism at the end of our session, which will translate into subsequent activities.

◊ Life

Life is the principle that governs the entire functioning of nature. It is the principle of expansion, movement, desire and material and psychological prosperity at the root of all evolution.

◊ The vibration

Prâna can always be perceived either in its vibratory nature or in its light nature. With a little practice, we can perceive the vibration. It flows like an eternal waterfall.

◊ The balance

Prâna is balance. It never brings excitement. But if we exceed our current capacities, we risk over-stimulating our nature. Because of this balancing quality, prâna heals and restores physical and psychological disorders.

◊ The light

By focusing on the light perception associated with prâna, we amplify it and can concentrate on the psychological and spiritual aspect of light.

◊ Fullness and bliss

We've talked about five characteristics of prâna: *vibration, life, light, balance and energy*. As we progress further, we discover a sixth, which is *fullness*. Concentrating on this aspect will amplify the experience. We discover an intense, refined enjoyment that overflows all the limits of our being, a rapture, an unknown bliss that is nonetheless not foreign to our nature.

The perception of prâna

At first, we imagine it, but sensation soon replaces imagination. The most direct method is to concentrate in the kumbhakas on the prâna within, first in the solar plexus, then in the belly space. It then becomes easy to arouse and feel it in any part of the body, then in the whole body. Other practices, such as belly bandhas, Ashwinî mudrâ or Kaki mudrâ, easily generate this sensation of prâna. Prâna is perceived visually as a luminosity in the body, as a vibration or radiant force. Without direct perception, prânâyâma and all vibratory disciplines, as well as the art of prâna manipulation, cannot claim to be fully effective.

Self-transformation through prâna obviously begins with its perception, whether physical or vibratory.

Kumbhaka is the best way to concentrate prâna.

We'll choose the rhythm **1 : 4 : 2** (5 : 20 : 10).

△ Inhale completely, with both nostrils, in 5 seconds, for example.

▲ Hold the breath for 20 seconds, perceiving and concentrating the prâna.

▽ Exhale in 10 seconds, directing the prâna into the defective organ with the representation of a luminous energy of health, balance and harmony.

The longer the breath, the more efficient you'll be.

You can practice in Ujjâyî.

♦ 1st stage: concentration on the chest

Start by feeling the prâna at chest level (prâna radiates and overflows beyond the skin),

♦ 2nd stage: concentrating on the stomach

♦ 3rd stage: concentration in the pelvis.

♦ 4th stage: concentration on prâna throughout the trunk, from the perineum to the throat.

♦ 5th stage: concentration on the perception of prâna throughout the body.

♦ 6th stage: concentration on the perception of prâna, either at belly level or for therapeutic use.

Going through the first five stages ensures that we are in an experience and not in a mental projection.

The chest space is AIR energy. The belly space is FIRE. The abdomen is WATER. The pelvic floor and legs are EARTH. By selecting them wisely, therapeutic properties are amplified.

Prâna that leaks and disintegrates is bad. Chaotic, uncontrolled, unpleasant prâna is bad. Prâna that is centered and concentrated is good. Prâna that is light, that radiates, is good. The prâna that concentrates thought, brings enthusiasm and confidence, is good. The prâna that brings fullness, gentleness, energy and strength is excellent. The prâna that soothes, balances and heals even before you ask it to, is excellent.

Moving on to higher rhythms

We can move on to the next rhythm once we've mastered it. We can think we've mastered a rhythm when we're comfortable with 14 successive breaths (or seven cycles in Nâdî Shodana) three days in a row.

If we've mastered the 5:20:10 rhythm, the next day we can practice 4 breaths in 6:24:12 and 6 breaths with the previous 5:20:10 rhythm. On subsequent days, we can add 2 breaths of the new 6:24:12 rhythm to each session, so as to make slow progress towards our new goal after several days.

Here are some tips on how to get the most out of prânâyâma:

> *In the Indian yogic tradition, prânâyâma includes breath retention. Ambition, haste, mental tension and bandhas practised incorrectly or not at all are the main sources of disorders caused by prânâyâma. To this can be added lack of preparation (warm-up).*
>
> *Prânâyâma is incompatible with medication, alcohol, drugs and, of course, tobacco. It is facilitated by all natural health factors. It must be practiced in a calm, harmonious environment and state of mind.*

For gifted students :

If you're exceptionally comfortable with apneas, you can try other higher rhythms.

They are :

1 : 6 : 4 : 1. 5 : 30 : 20 : 5. 6 : 36 : 24 : 6
1 : 8 : 6 : 1. 5 : 40 : 30 : 5. 6 : 48 : 36 : 6

In which you can later lay Shunyaka.

1 : 6 : 4 : 2. 5 : 30 : 20 : 10. 6 : 36 : 24 : 12
1 : 8 : 6 : 2. 5 : 40 : 30 : 10. 6 : 48 : 36 : 12

You need to be comfortable with both breath and concentration. However, you will find that concentration on prâna or on a subtle center greatly facilitates breath retention. Conversely, the longer you hold the breath, the longer and deeper you can experience prâna.

There is no need to go beyond this in a meditation orientation. The higher rhythms presented above imply daily practice and a strong commitment. The dedication of one hour a day is minimal. Not to mention the practice of postures and meditation itself.

On the other hand, you can consider prânâyâma as a meditation practice, and replace meditations with short concentrations or relaxations and centering in life. Then learn to consider prâna in its universal or spiritual dimension, and to perceive it everywhere – especially in natural atmospheres.

The rhythms of shunyaka

The basic rhythms of prânâyâma with Shunyaka, empty retention, are :

◆ 1st stage: equalize inspiration and exhalation
◆ 2nd stage: double the exhalation **(1:2)**; for example 4:8
◆ 3rd stage: introduction of shunyaka **(1 : 1 : 1)**; for example, triangular empty breathing 8 (inhale) : 8 (exhale) : 8 (shunyaka)
◆ 4th stage: rhythm **(1 : 2 : 2)**; for example 6 : 12 : 12
◆ 5th stage: rhythm **(1 : 2 : 3)**; for example 6 : 12 : 18
◆ 6th stage: rhythm **(1 : 2 : 4)**; for example 6 : 12 : 24 or 8 : 16 : 32. After this rhythm comes the :
◆ 7th stage: rhythm **(1 : 2 : 6)**; for example 6 : 12 : 36

If we choose to practice not for internalization, but for the growth of strength-consciousness, we add Uddîyâna bandha. *Uddîyâna bandha* can be introduced from the fifth stage onwards. At first, it does not need to be performed thoroughly.

N° 85 – PRÂNÂYÂMA WITH SHUNYAKA ★★★

There are two types of prânâyâmas with shunyaka. The first is associated with short retentions, without bandhas, particularly without Uddîyâna bandha. It is one of the practices that bring feminine prâna and internalization.

The second type is performed with bandhas, particularly Uddîyâna. With empty lungs, it creates a strong depression and reinforces the individual's internal energy and consciousness-strength. It is related to male prâna, but is more interiorizing than prânâyâma with kumbhaka, and its effects are more spiritual. It contributes to the awakening of the Kundalinî. The first type is described in Subtle Breathing (chapter 11).

This chapter deals with the second type.

We'll take the rhythm **1 : 2 : 3** (6 : 12 : 18)

△ Inhale completely, in 6 seconds, for example.

▲ Hold your breath for 1 second.

▽ Exhale in 12 seconds with a 1/2 Mûla bandha, which you will also keep during empty retention.

▼ Hold the empty breath for 18 seconds, closing the glottis with full Mûla bandha.

Breathe out a little to unblock the breath, remove the Mûla bandha, then breathe in again in 6 seconds...

From 20 seconds in the shunyaka, integrate the two bandhas: Jâlandhara and Mûla bandha into the vacuum retention.

△ Inhale completely, in 5 seconds, for example.

▲ Hold your breath for 1 second.

▽ Exhale in 10 seconds and take the Jâlandhara bandha, then the Mûla bandha, which you will hold for the duration of the vacuum retention.

▼ Hold the empty breath for 15 seconds, closing the glottis and keeping the Mûla bandha tight.

△ Exhale a little to unblock the breath, raise the head and remove the Mûla bandha, then inhale again in 5 seconds...

N° 86 – PRÂNÂYÂMA WITH THE THREE BANDHAS ★★★

The three bandhas are *Jâlandhara bandha*, for the throat, *Mûla bandha* for the pelvic floor and *Uddîyâna bandha* for the abdomen.

△ Inhale completely, in 5 seconds, for example.

Hold your breath for 1 second.

▽ Exhale in 10 seconds, then, in order, bend your head and take the Jâlandhara bandha, then press with your hands on your thighs to take the Uddîyâna bandha, then take the Mûla bandha. These are the three bandhas you'll hold for the duration of the empty retention.

▼ Hold the empty breath for 15 seconds, closing the glottis tightly, with the 3 bandhas.

△ At the end of shunyaka, release, in the reverse order in which you took them: Mûla bandha, then Uddîyâna (release the belly), then Jâland-hara (raise the head). Exhale a little to release the breath, then inhale again quietly over 5 seconds...

This prânâyâma, along with the Uddîyâna bandha, is the most powerful; it is also the most difficult to master.

The 15-second duration chosen here is suggested for learning to master the technique.

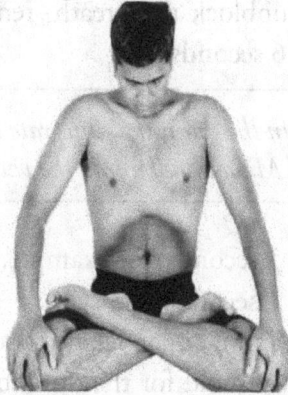

The three bandhas in shunyaka

Concentration in retention areas

Prânâyâma with Kumbhaka requires inflexible concentration, even more so than in the early stages of meditation. Thoughts and distractions are forbidden. Concentrate on relaxing the eyes, shoulders and mind, and on the bandhas.

> *The practice of kumbhaka is:*
> ♦ *Intense contraction of the bandhas,*
> ♦ *Deep relaxation of head, shoulders and mind.*
> ♦ *An unwavering concentration of consciousness.*

Thereafter, the adept will adopt concentration during long retentions, particularly Kumbhaka.

The main concentrations we recommend are :
◊ The whole body feels like a block, a unit

◊ Left/right balancing

◊ The stability of prâna, citta or the mind

◊ Prâna perception (see therapeutic prânâyâma)

◊ The 5 centers for meditation (Sahasrâra, Âjnâ, Anahâta, Mûlâdhâra or Sushumnâ)

◊ Consciousness-strength, in relation to our spiritual individuality, which we associate with centering, or better still, with Sushumnâ.

◊ The seven chakras, with one chakra per nâdî Shodana cycle, i.e. 2 kumbhakas per chakra. In this case, we'll be practicing seven cycles.

We advise against concentrating on a single chakra during all kumbhakas. This would inevitably lead to the overdynamization of one part of our nature, to the detriment of a harmonious and balanced method of development.

Let's not forget the power of kumbhaka and prâna concentration. And we know that safeguard lies in controlled progressiveness. Let's cultivate common sense, calm, balance, moderation and patience. Beware of ambition and impatient ego.

Immobility and stability, concentration, inner strength, self-control, equanimity, mastery over all psychological movements (thoughts, images, sensations, emotions, etc.) are all born of the stability of citta, but are undoubtedly destroyed by excess and loss of prâna mastery.

XIII
AWAKENING THE CHAKRAS
THROUGH PRÂNÂYÂMA

Âjnâ: Guide and Initiator

In the ancient yoga tradition, Conscious Being, called *Purusha* in San-skrit, and Nature, *Prakriti*, are the two sides of spiritual reality manifested in the universe. In their individual forms, *Purusha*, the Conscious Being, signifies the Soul, and *Prakriti* represents the nature of the human being. Sri Aurobindo describes the Conscious Being as follows:

> *The conscious Being, Purusha, is the Self as generator, witness, supporter, enjoyer and Master of forms and works. [...] Purusha is present in all planes: there is a physical purusha, a vital purusha and a mental puru-sha, which is the guide of life and the body, as the Upanishad says...*

The Mental Conscious Being, the Soul's delegate in the human being, has five roles:

◊ Seeking knowledge and truth,
◊ Making human beings conscious,
◊ Guide and direct it,
◊ Centralizing and structuring the individual
◊ Organizing indoor and outdoor living.

The Conscious Being is located at Âjnâ. This makes it the first chakra to be awakened and the main place for our centering. It is the chakra that can bring us security in our inner and outer journey.

Transforming the citta and awakening the chakras with prânâyâma

Breath-holding stabilizes the citta and focuses the consciousness-strength. This creates the ideal conditions for chakra stimulation.

The chakras used for meditation are :

◊ Âjnâ chakra, the chakra of mental awareness,

◊ Anâhata chakra, for vital awareness and the deep heart,

◊ Mûlâdhâra chakra, the base chakra, in relation to Sushumnâ, the central channel and Kundalini,

◊ Sahasrâra, the Lotus of a Thousand Petals, above the head, which opens to the Divine above and to the Higher Mind.

◊ We can add Sushumnâ, the central channel through which the human being is connected to universal energy.

All these centers are gateways to deep consciousness, linked to the spiritual dimension of the human being.

Each chakra has a frontal counterpart, more in touch with external life, and a dorsal part, more subconscious.

Citta is the energetic and psychological ground, described as the substance of consciousness[1]. All natural movements, thoughts, images, emotions and sensations are formed from this material. So it's easy to understand that working on this "soil" of consciousness is immensely productive, because it can transform all natural movements.

That's why we'll be working on the chakras, which have their subtle seat in the spine, on their frontal counterpart and on the chakra citta.

The most important of all, – the closest, the least encumbered by subconscious impressions and because it represents in our nature the conscious Being and guide, is Âjnâ chakra, with its frontal counterpart, Bhrûmadhya, its space (called Chidâkash) and its citta.

Bhrûmadhya

(N° 48) – THE PRACTICE OF ASHWINÎ MUDRÂ AND BHRÛMADHYA ★★★

We have already seen the practice of Ashwinî mudrâ. This mudrâ is of particular interest here because it naturally stimulates Bhrûmadhya. This is why, during the *mudrâ*, focus your attention on this point in the middle of the forehead. After the mudrâ, as we have seen, concentrate

---

1. The substance of the mental, vital and subtle physical is citta, just as the substance of the body is matter.

with your eyes closed on the inner feeling of prâna in the body, then on Bhrûmadhya.

(N° 29) – KAPÂLABHÂTI AND BHRÛMADHYA

Kapâlabhâti naturally stimulates the frontal part of the brain. When its execution becomes automatic, without effort, adopt this concentration at the same time on Bhrûmadhya and prolong it after the prânâyâma.

N° 87 – SQUARE BREATHING AND BHRÛMADHYA ★★★

Begin square breathing, in *Ujjâyî*, gradually lengthening and regulating the breath.

Then perform *Mûla bandha* during both breath-holds, full and empty. Release the bandha on the inhale and exhale.

Finally, add concentration on *Bhrûmadhya* in both retentions. As you inhale and exhale, concentrate on the uniformity of sound in *Ujjâyî*.

In both retentions, concentrate on muscular and mental relaxation, the contraction of the base, *Mûla bandha*, and on *Bhrûmadhya*. With practice, your mind will quickly integrate these different techniques and practice will become easy and enjoyable.

△ Inhale with Ujjâyî.

▲ Kumbhaka: concentration in Bhrûmadhya + *Mûla bandha*.

▽ Exhale with Ujjâyî.

▼ Shunyaka: concentration in Bhrûmadhya + *Mûla bandha*.

Then prolong concentration on Bhrûmadhya without worrying about breathing.

The mind is calmed, then focused and stabilized.

During the practice of Kâpâlabhâti, concentrate on the Bhrûmadhya energy center, in the middle of the forehead, with half a *Mûla bandha*.

Âjnâ chakra

N° 88 – KAPÂLABHÂTI AND ÂJNÂ ★★★

In the same way as in the above exercise, concentrate on Âjnâ in the empty retention that follows Kapâlabhâti. Don't hesitate to prolong this concentration even after you've normalized your breathing. Gradually build up to three cycles.

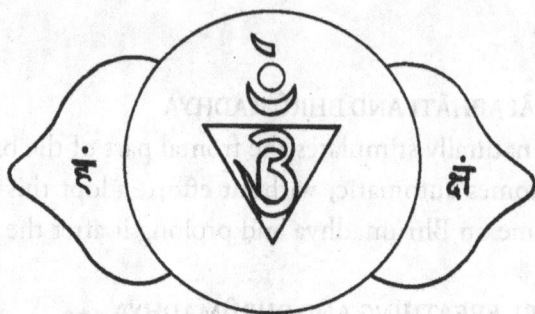

Âjnâ chakra

N° 89 – TRIANGULAR BREATHING (KUMBHAKA) AND ÂJNÂ ★★★

Adopt a comfortable position, suitable for prânâyâma, and begin triangular breathing with kumbhaka.

△ Inhale in 8 seconds, for example.

▲ Kumbhaka in 8 seconds: concentration at Âjnâ + 1/2 *Mûla bandha*.

▽ Exhale in 8 seconds.

Start with concentration on Âjnâ only in full-lung retention for about ten breaths, then generalize concentration on Âjnâ in all three beats.

Then extend the internalization to Âjnâ without worrying about breathing.

Don't hesitate to repeat the prânâyâma if concentration wanes.

N° 90 – SAMATÂ PRÂNÂYÂMA AND ÂJNÂ

Merging Samatâ prânâyâma and concentration on Âjnâ.

Breathing should be slow, regular, continuous, even and subtle. Take inspiration from exercise N° 74, The perfect curve.

N° 91 – SAMAVRITTI PRÂNÂYÂMA AND ÂJNÂ ★★★

Settle into the position of concentration.

Then begin the practice of square breathing, in Ujjâyî.

When you've reached your cruising speed, introduce *Mûla bandha*, the contraction of the base, into the inhale, exhale and empty retention.

Then, once you've mastered prânâyâma with *Mûla bandha*, you can add concentration on Âjnâ.

N° 92 – PRÂNÂYÂMA OF THE BEE AND ÂJNÂ ★★★

Bhrâmarî prânâyâma, the Bee Breath, consists in emitting a buzzing nasal sound, with ears and mouth closed, as you exhale. If you've mastered it, emit the high-pitched sound on the inhale as well.

Close your eyes and make this nasal sound, resonating in the center of the Âjnâ chakra.

Then stay inside Âjnâ to listen to the subtle sounds or the sound of silence.

N° 93 – SHÂMBAVÎ MUDRÂ AND ÂJNÂ ★★★

This mudra strongly stimulates the Ajna chakra.

Stare at the Shâmbavî[1] mudrâ for a few moments, then relax your eyes and internalize in the Ajnâ chakra. This constitutes a cycle. Perform several cycles, gradually lengthening your concentration.

In India, the assiduous practice of this mudrâ can lead to a Kundalinî awakening or to the highest stages of meditation.

Other chakras

N° 94 – TRIANGULAR PRÂNÂYÂMA (SHUNYAKA) + MÛLÂDHÂRA CONCENTRATION ★★★

Adopt a comfortable position, suitable for prânâyâma, and begin triangular breathing with Shunyaka.

△ Inhale in 8 seconds, for example.

▽ Exhale in 8 seconds.

▼ Shunyaka in 8 seconds: concentration in Mûlâdhâra + 1/2 *Mûla bandha* + 1/2 *Uddîyâna bandha*.

Start with concentration on Mûlâdhâra only in empty retention for a few breaths, then generalize concentration on Mûlâdhâra in all three beats.

Then prolong the internalization in Mûlâdhâra without worrying about breathing.

Don't hesitate to repeat the prânâyâma if concentration wanes, centering on Mûlâdhâra.

Alternate prânâyâma and static concentration on Mûlâdhâra.

---

1. Shâmbavî mudrâ : see N° 42

You can also choose to concentrate on Sushumnâ, which you visualize as a thin, straight, vertical column of light at spinal level. Carefully balance the 2 hemispheres.

Anâhata, the Heart chakra

If you choose the heart chakra, Anâhata, remove the 1/2 *Uddîyâna bandha*.

Samatâ prânâyâma or the Bee are also ideal for concentration on the heart chakra.

XIV
THE STABILITY OF
MENTAL *CITTA*

The substance of consciousness, citta

"Citta is the substance of the mental-vital-physical triple consciousness from which arise the movements of thought, emotion, sensation, impulse, etc." – Sri Aurobindo, *The Yoga Guide*

Citta is the substance of consciousness, the vibratory mind, the mind-substance.

But it can also be represented in psychological terms, and as such is the reservoir of all psychological impressions, whether conscious, subconscious or subliminal. In this case, we'll approach it primarily in the form of atmospheres, but also images and thoughts.

The citta is therefore the substance of the psyche and the reservoir of all past impressions; it thus corresponds to total memory. Insofar as it is recognized as holotropic, citta is comparable to the homeopathic or naturopathic notion of "terrain. Even so, it's not wrong, and it can sometimes be interesting, to distinguish between mental citta, vital or emotional citta and subtle physical citta.

The properties of the citta depend on its content, which changes with its depth and with the representation we choose. Indeed, deep within us, the citta houses both the unconscious[1] (or subconscious) and the sub-

1. Sri Aurobindo considers Freud's description of the Unconscious to be narrow, with an exaggeration of certain sides and a total ignorance of the existence of any luminous part in the human being (subliminal or supraconscious). The problem, moreover, lies not in the limitation of knowledge, but in the pride and arrogance that can arise from the accumulation of knowledge. For science to open a new chapter,

liminal described by Sri Aurobindo.

The subliminal corresponds to our deepest nature (mental, vital or physical); it is conscious and closer to the vast universal nature and eternal realities the closer it gets to the Divine within.

The subconscious, on the other hand, is always a low-awareness environment. It expresses the confusion and suffering of physical, vital and mental memories, situations of intense fear, frustration or disappointment, failures, dead-ends or denials of identity, life and love. It therefore also represents all our resistance, ill will, conditioning and inertia to living, opening up and progressing. The subconscious corresponds to all the "impressionsfrom the past that we haven't assimilated, and often originates in early childhood and our previous lives.

But this subconscious, Sri Aurobindo tells us, is only a small part of our deeper nature. Through self-transformation, it unravels and dissolves as we move closer to our true being, our center, the heart of our Heart.

On the surface, our mental citta is obscure, restless, chaotic, narrow and rigid, unconscious, and at first resembles a tiny, stuffy room. This is so because our surface citta rests on its subconscious foundations and the omnipresence of the ego. In the yogi, the surface citta is transformed. It is luminous, peaceful and yet always full of energy; it expresses spaciousness, plasticity, gentleness, objectless bliss and natural, permanent vigilance.

We can penetrate this subtle substance through internalization. Conscious, controlled internalization will reveal a calm environment that brings us states of concentration, stability, alertness, breadth, openness, contentment and ease.

On the surface, thoughts and images form in the citta; deeper down, thoughts disappear and images and sensations take center stage. In deeper internalization, images and sensations disappear or become universalized. Calm deepens, followed by immobility and stability. The density of our being increases with depth: the density of our substance, the intensity of our consciousness, the revelation of our existence.

it requires the sacrifice of many pioneers and the stubbornness of a few researchers whose quest for knowledge is above suspicion.

> *In classical meditation, citta stability is achieved through prolonged concen-*
> *tration. Here, we experiment with vibratory methods.*

N° 95 – DISCOVERING CITTA ★★★

The notion of subtle substance is not foreign to us. It reflects an evolu-tion from material density to an increasingly fluid and ethereal state. We find it hard to move through the mud of a pond, but easier to move through water when we swim underwater. Even more fluid, we experi-ence the fog and atmosphere that surrounds us and which we breathe.

Taking the experiment a step further, if we look up at the cloudless sky or at the space in front of us, we can perceive tiny bright dots in motion. Similarly, the various gases and constituents of the atmosphere can be revealed in the dark by a beam of light, or by breath on a cold day. The same applies to the inner space of the head, Chidâkâsh. Its substance is revealed to us by luminous or coloured movements and by a different vibratory activity according to our inner states. In certain cases, such as anger or other strong emotions, the citta in the head is violently agitated in all directions.

Enter the inner space of your head, Chidâkâsh, close your eyes and imagine this space as a fog or an infinite number of small dots, more or less luminous, more or less dense or mobile. Rapidly, if you continue to concentrate on the substance, you will begin to perceive impressions of movement, different luminous intensities and the beginnings of subtle, fluctuating, ever-changing forms. This is the expression of citta.

Remember that by changing your representation, you can access Chidâkâsh as a space or as a citta.

> *The representation of citta is that of a substance.*
> *The representation of prâna is a luminous fluid in itself.*

Citta stability and soul equality

Equality of soul is a fundamental quality that we must cultivate if we are to progress in meditation. It's the ability to renounce judgment and consider all things with equal attention. It is psychologically based on non-reaction and integration, the opposite of exclusion. Integration is associated with the expansion of consciousness.

From a psychological point of view, citta stability is associated with soul equality.

N° 96 – SAMATÂ PRÂNÂYÂMA AND THE STABILITY OF CITTA

Samatâ prânâyâma is a subtle breathing technique in which we seek a uniform flow of breath on both the inhalation and exhalation sides, an equalization of the two beats of the breath, with maximum lengthening and slowness. Here, we add Ujjâyî prânâyâma.

Uniformity of breath leads to citta immobility, then stability.

N° 97 – KAPÂLABHÂTI AND THE STABILITY OF CITTA ★★★

Practice Kapâlabhâti progressively until you are able to hold 3 cycles of 50 breaths, interspersed with an empty suspension. Concentrate on Chidâkâsh and enter the immobility and stability of the head citta.

N° 98 – KAPÂLABHÂTI, SHÂMBAVÎ AND MÛLA BANDHA ★★★

After Kâpâlabhâti, perform an empty retention by adding *Shâmbavî* and *Mûla bandhas*. Relax your eyes and mind before continuing with another cycle.

Perform three cycles, then concentrate on the stability of the citta in the head.

N° 99 – EMPTY BREATH RETENTION AND PSYCHIC STABILITY

Breath retention with full (kumbhaka) or empty (shunyaka) lungs leads to citta stability. Adopt the triangular empty breath or Samatâ prânâyâma with two suspensions of breath without closing the glottis. Adopt the rhythm 1 : 2 : 1 : 2, as for example 4 : 8 : 4 : 8. Concentrate on the stability of the citta in the 2 suspensions.

N° 100 – STABILITY THROUGH SHUNYAKA AND BANDHAS ★★★

Practice triangular breathing, with shunyaka, vacuum retention.

When the rhythm is well established, add *Mûla bandha* and half an *Uddîyâna* to the empty retention. Don't force the bandhas at all. On the contrary, practice them half-heartedly. Concentrate on shunyaka stability. If necessary, alternate from time to time with triangular breathing without bandhas.

N° 101 – STABILITY THROUGH KUMBHAKA AND BANDHAS ★★★

Start the triangular breathing with kumbhaka, for example 8 : 8 : 8. After a few moments, add *Mûla bandha*, the contraction of the base in the retention of the breath, then concentration on the immobility and stability of the citta.

N° 102 – DISCOVERING MENTAL CITTA THROUGH SHÂMBAVÎ MUDRÂ

Practice *Shâmbavî mudrâ* very gradually, taking care to balance left and right vision and to relax the mind and eyes during the practice. Alternate mudrâ and Chidâkâsh visualization several times. *Shâmbavî mudrâ* makes the citta luminous and colorful, revealing the inner space.

We can also experience citta and chidâkâsh by pressing on our eyes with closed eyelids, or by practicing palming with concentration on inner space. So here are 3 different ways of experiencing citta and Chidâkâsh.

N° 103 – SQUARE BREATHING AND SHÂMBAVÎ MUDRÂ ★★★

Start the breath in Ujjâyî, and when it's easy, add *Shâmbavî mudrâ* to the full-lung retention (kumbhaka). In Kumbhaka, relax the neck and shoulders, and in the other breaths, relax the eyes in particular.

N° 104 – SHUNYAKA AND SHÂMBAVÎ MUDRÂ ★★★

In triangular breathing with empty retention, combine *Shâmbavî mudrâ and Mûla bandha* in retention. Alternate with concentration on the stability of the citta, in which you relax your eyes.

Shâmbavî mudrâ and *Mûla bandha* reinforce each other.

N° 105 – TRIBANDHA AND SHÂMBAVÎ MUDRÂ ★★★

Exhale fully and hold the breath in shunyaka to practice the *Mahâ bandha*, also called *Tribandha* because it's made up of the 3 bandhas: *Jâlandhara, Uddîyâna and Mûla bandhas*. You can amplify the effects even further by adding *Shâmbavî mudrâ*. Alternate this bandha with static concentration on stability.

(N° 46) – AKASHI MUDRÂ ★★★

△ Inhaling gently in Ujjâyî, slowly move your head backwards, without excess. Hold it in this position and practice Ujjâyî prânâyâma, adding *Khecarî mudrâ*, with the tongue folded over the upper palate, and *Shâmbavî mudrâ*.

In this position, concentrate on the Âjnâ chakra. Take a few deep breaths. Then slowly bring the head back, remove all bandhas and mudrâs and remain internalized.

Then concentrate on keeping the citta stable in this position for a few moments, without worrying about breathing, and eventually repeat the whole process. By adding a cycle to each session, you can go up to 5 cycles.

Proceed with caution. If you feel dizzy, contract the *Mûla bandha* strongly and return. If you can't avoid dizziness, abandon the practice.

Empty breath retention, Shunyaka, prânâyâma of the Bee and practices with Shâmbavî mudrâ are ideal for concentration on Âjnâ or the Thousand-Petalled Lotus above the head. We'll look at other practices in subsequent chapters.

We'll be perfecting citta stability and soul equality in the next section on mental silence.

XV
INTRODUCTION TO INNER
SPACE INTERIOR: *CHIDÂKASH*

The inner space, *Chidâkash*

Chidâkash dhâranâ is a tantric discipline based on the vision of the screen and inner space.

By this we mean a visual concentration on what we see when our eyes are closed in the head space. By considering these visual impressions in front of us, we can imagine the inner cavity of the forehead as a screen or space.

N° 106 – INTERIOR SPACE IN PALMING ★★★

Rub your palms vigorously together for a few moments to energize them, then apply them in a dome shape to each of your eyes, without touching them and eliminating the passage of light. Close your eyes, letting them absorb all the vitality of your hands, and concentrate on seeing the darkness and relaxing your eyes and mind.

Repeat the whole process once or twice.

N° 107 – INNER SPACE WITH BHOOCHARÎ MUDRÂ1, THE MUDRÂ OF EMPTINESS ★★★

Hold your arm out in front of you, close your hand and lift your thumb. Then concentrate for a few moments on the thumbnail and remove your hand. Then keep your mind on the perception of this point in the void

---

1. Bhoochari mudrâ : see N° 39.

in front of you and expand your visual perception to the whole space in front of you, as large as possible, without locking your gaze on any object.

Practice this mudrâ with your eyes open, and become aware of the empty space in front of you, without hanging any object, then close your eyes and continue to visualize and feel this same space inside *Chidâkâsh*.

N° 108 – FRONTAL SPACE AFTER KÂPÂLABHÂTI

Practice Kapâlabhâti prânâyâma, 30 to 50 breaths, then, in empty retention, concentrate visually on the screen or frontal space of Chidâkâsh. Concentrate on what you see with your eyes closed, without images or thoughts. Prolong this concentration for a few moments before starting another series.

VARIANT: KAPÂLABHÂTI AND THE FAR FRONT SPACE

You can also take advantage of the vacuum retention that follows the breathing of the Bellows to visualize the distant frontal space. In this exercise, try to push the screen or frontal space back about 50 cm, using your imagination.

N° 109 – KAPÂLABHÂTI AND THE UPPER HEAD SPACE

Take advantage of the empty-lung retention that follows Kapâlabhâti practice to concentrate on visualizing the inner space in the upper part of the head at forehead level, just below the top of the skull. Visualize omnidirectional space by positioning yourself at this level.

Prolong this concentration for a few moments after the prânâyâma.

N° 110 – COMPLETE CHIDÂKÂSH AFTER KAPÂLABHÂTI ★★★

After making the gussets, during vacuum retention, visualize the headspace in all directions.

Prolong this concentration for a few moments after the prânâyâma.

N° 111 – THE FAR FRONT SPACE AND THE SQUARE-BREATHING BACK SPACE

Practice square breathing. Then close your eyes and go inside your head.

△▲ Inhale and kumbhaka: visualize the frontal space beyond the forehead at 50 cm.

▽▼ Exhalation and shunyaka: visualization of rear space.

Alternatively, you can choose to double the retention time in relation to the duration of the inhale or exhale. This would give, for example, 5–10–5–10 with 5 seconds for the inhale and exhale, and 10 seconds for both retentions.

Prolong this concentration for a few moments after the prânâyâma.

TRIANGULAR BREATHING VARIANT

Practice empty triangular breathing. Then close your eyes and go inside your head.

△ Inhale: visualize the frontal space.

▽ Exhale: visualize the back space.

▼ Suspend the empty breath and maintain concentration on the back space.

Prolong this concentration for a few moments after the prânâyâma.

This breathing generates great inner calm.

Nº 112 – CHIDÂKASH WITH SQUARE BREATHING

Practice square breathing. Then close your eyes and go inside your head.

In the retentions, visualize the space inside the head in all directions.

Prolong this concentration for a few moments after the prânâyâma.

XVI
INTRODUCTION TO
THOUGHT CONTROL

Thought control through breathing

N° 113 – BHOOCHARÎ MUDRÂ1 AND THOUGHTS ★★★

Chidâkâsh brings spatial emptiness, the emptiness of substance; *Bhoochari mudrâ*, psychological emptiness.

Concentrate first on the empty, content-free **spot**, first with your eyes open, then with your eyes closed. Then do the same with the largest possible empty **space.** Continue with your eyes closed.

Whenever a thought enters your mind, return to emptiness without reaction. In this way, develop your equanimity.

It's a particularly effective exercise.

N° 114 – SQUARE BREATHING AND THOUGHTS ★★★

Settle into the position of concentration. Then begin the practice of square breathing.

When you have reached your cruising level, introduce Mûla bandha, the contraction of the base, into both retentions.

While continuing the square breathing, gather your concentration, then concentrate in Chidâkâsh and inner vigilance. Don't allow thoughts to come in.

After a while, finish your breathing exercise and continue the thought control for another ten minutes.

---

1. Bhoochari mudrâ: see N° 39 and N° 107.

N° 115 – BRAIN BALANCING AND THOUGHTS ★★★

Focus on the brain and separate the left brain from the right.

Begin the Ujjâyî breath and equalize the duration of the inhalation and exhalation.

△ Inhale: visualize and feel the left brain.

▽ Exhale: visualize and feel the right brain.

△ Inhale: visualize and feel the right brain.

▽ Exhale: visualize and feel the left brain.

This constitutes a cycle. Practice about ten cycles.

Then place yourself in the center of Chidâkâsh and observe the witnessing thoughts.

If the thoughts keep coming back, repeat the brain rebalancing exercise, then return to the thought witness.

N° 116 – SAMATÂ PRÂNÂYÂMA AND THOUGHTS ★★★

Practice Samatâ prânâyâma by equalizing the inhale and exhale.

At the same time, witness your thoughts.

After a while, let go of breath control while continuing to observe your thoughts.

N° 117 – SÂVITRÎ PRÂNÂYÂMA AND SELF-AWARENESS ★★★

Center yourself in Âjnâ and start the rectangular or triangular empty breath. Once you've mastered the rhythm, combine it with a short concentration on self-awareness or presence in the retention(s).

Then concentrate on Chidâkâsh in the state of non-thought and inner vigilance.

XVII
INTRODUCTION TO KRIYÂS

The kriyâ technique

Kriyâ is a technique of conscious prâna manipulation, combined with concentration, in the subtle physical or prânic body. This manipulation can take several forms:

The path. This consists in creating a movement of prâna between one energy point and another, or a zone of the prânic body. This is the most common method.

The "dynamic relationship" between two energy points or zones to achieve an enriched fusion of the "dynamic duality type, defined as two points separated yet remaining unified or fused.

Manipulating the citta: rebalancing, expanding, expanding/contracting or elevating it.

A combination of mudrâs and bandhas, prânâyâma and concentration.

Movement breaks the rigidity of being, characterized by ego and conditioning. Inner disciplines that integrate movement have in common that they promote receptivity and facilitate concentration.

This movement of the prâna is initially carried out by will and imagination, in synchronization with the breath. It may also be accompanied by a mantra, visualization, a particular posture, breath-holding, mudras and bandhas, or concentration on one or more energy centers or zones (chakras).

The aim of kriyâ is to manipulate prâna and citta; this brings about a change in the practitioner's consciousness and inner condition.

The most powerful form of kriyâ occurs when you actually feel prâna in motion. It is quickly followed by the spontaneous, automatic movement of prâna. This phenomenon is similar in nature to the automatic repetition of a mantra.

We'll start with a few rebalancing kriyâs.

Some rebalancing

Dynamic Duality (D/D) is a technique for creating relationships between two energy centers, using the breath as a support.

△ Inhale and focus on center A.

▽ Exhale and focus on center B.

△ Inhale and focus on center B.

▽ Exhale and focus on center A.

This constitutes a cycle.

Kriyâ is linked to prâna and consciousness. In D/D, as in kriyâ, the right way to proceed is to practice as if the exercise would never end, to situate oneself outside time. On the other hand, unlike kriyâ, in D/D there is no movement. The Dynamic Duality technique is nevertheless easier.

For these practices, adopt the Samatâ prânâyâma (N° 65).

N° 118 – D/D: NECK / FOREHEAD

The two parts of the head, frontal and occipital, correspond to two opposite polarities of internal energy; they also correspond to the oldest part of evolution (back and deep) and the most recent (frontal and cortical).

Equalizing these two zones eliminates mental saturation and reconnects us to the deeper dimension of the body.

The effect of any rebalancing is to remove tension and reactivate blocked forces and circuits.

△ Inhale, concentrating on the whole forehead.

▽ Exhale, focusing on the back of the head and the nape of the neck.

△ Inhale, remaining on the back of the head.

▽ Exhale with forehead centered.

Practice a minimum of ten cycles, then remain relaxed and receptive for a few moments.

N° 119 – D/D : NECK / SOLAR PLEXUS

Certain points or areas of the body can be matched to create an energetic and psychic rebalancing. Remember that breathing must be regular, slow and silent. However, we can also practice *Ujjâyî* (cf. N° 19) with a soft sound which must be perfectly audible to the practitioner, but inaudible to others in the vicinity. In *Ujjâyî*, the softer the sound, the greater the desire for interiorization. In all cases, concentrate on the uniformity of the sound.

This exercise in particular removes nervous tension.

△ Inhale slowly and concentrate on the back of the neck and the back of the head.

▽ Exhale and concentrate on the solar plexus.

△ Inhale and concentrate on the solar plexus.

▽ Exhale and return to the nape of the neck and the back of the head.

Practice 5 to 10 cycles.

Relax and center yourself.

If you wish to deepen your experience, repeat a series of cycles.

Generally speaking, you can practice with your eyes open or closed. If your attention deepens, close your eyes, and if you need to undertake a dynamic activity afterwards, finish with a series of several cycles with your eyes open.

N° 120 – D/D: SKULL + PERINEUM

△ Inhale slowly and concentrate on the upper part of the skull.

▽ Exhale and concentrate on the perineum.

△ Inhale and concentrate on the perineum.

▽ Exhale and return to the top of the skull.

Practice 5 to 10 cycles. Then center yourself.

The deep mind and inner vigilance

As we saw in Chapter 13, *Âjnâ, The Guide and Initiator*, the Âjnâ chakra is a priority for development, particularly because of the strength of our subconscious. In fact, the Heart chakra is often highly charged with traumas linked to individuality (e.g. non-recognition in childhood) and love (e.g. the loss of a loved one), which are among the most difficult traumas.

The development of conscious Being in Âjnâ is even more necessary in a path of Kundalinî awakening.

We need first to grow our capacity for awareness, to witness and to ensure the inner guidance of Conscious Being.

N° 121 – KRIYÂ: BHRÛMADHYA AND FRONTAL SPACE ★★★

△ With eyes closed, raise the breath on the inhale, from the nostrils to Bhrûmadhya, in the middle of the forehead.

▽ As you exhale, visualize the frontal space in front of you from this point.

As usual, practice a series of cycles, then concentrate.

N° 122 – KRIYÂ: NOSTRILS ←→ BHRÛMADHYA (ANULOMA VILOMA) (front) ★★★

Bhrûmadhya

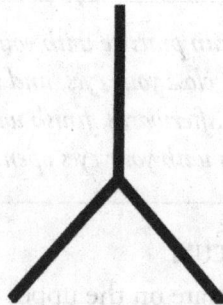

Left nostril Right nostril

△ Inhale through the left nostril, raising the subtle breath to Bhrûmadhya.

▽ Exhale and slowly bring Bhrûmadhya's prâna down towards the right nostril.

△ As you inhale, raise the breath through the right nostril to Bhrûmadhya.

▽ Exhaling, descend the passage to the left.

N° 123 – KRIYÂ: ANULOMA VILOMA: NOSTRILS ↔ BRAHMARANDHRA (front) ★★★

Compare this kriyâ with the previous one.

△ Inhale regularly and raise the prâna in the left nostril towards Bhrû-madhya, then continue the frontal circuit to Brahmarandhra, at the top of the head.

▽ Exhale slowly and descend through the right nostril.

△ Inhale and rise again to Brahmarandhra through the right nostril.

▽ Exhale and descend through the left nostril.

Feel free to suspend your breath for a second or two in Brahmarandhra before exhaling.

N° 124 – KRIYÂ: ANULOMA VILOMA AND ÂJNÂ ★★★

Practice alternating breathing without hands for a few moments, until it becomes regular. Then continue in this way, visualizing a subtle channel between the nostril and Âjnâ in the head.

△ Inhale through the left nostril and lead the subtle breath to Âjnâ.

▽ Exhale and lead Âjnâ's prâna to the right nostril.

△ Inhale through the right nostril as far as Âjnâ.

▽ Exhale from Âjnâ to the left nostril.

Continue in this way, then internalize Âjnâ.

N° 125 – KRIYÂ: THE INNER SURFACE OF THE FOREHEAD

△ Inhale slowly through Bhrûmadhya, the point in the middle of the forehead, and lead the prâna into the inner space of the head.

▽ Exhale just as slowly and evenly, and discover the inner surface of the forehead, which curves from the eyes to the top of the skull.

Practice 12 cycles or more, then concentrate for a few moments on the screen or frontal space that rises to the top of the skull.

N° 126 – KRIYÂ: INTERNAL SKULL SCANNING ★★★

△ Inhale slowly, in Samatâ prânâyâma[1] or in Ujjâyî, visualizing in a sweeping movement the entire inner surface of the forehead and skull upwards, then backwards to the nape of the neck.

1. Samatâ prânâyâma (N° 45). We can practice it with Ujjâyî, if we're looking for internalization, or without Ujjâyî if we're looking for contact with prâna.

▽ Exhale, visualizing and tactilely feeling the inner surface of the skull, from the nape of the neck to the forehead.

Initially, proceed in stages:

On your first breath, raise the entire inner surface of your forehead and then lower it back down to your nostrils as you exhale.

On the 2nd breath, go over the inner surface to the top of the skull.

At 3°, continue to the back of the skull and return to the exhalation at Trikutî.

Practice 12 cycles of complete kriyâ, then stand still and contemplate the entire inner surface of the skull, accentuating inner vigilance.

N° 127 – KRIYÂ: NOSTRILS ↔ BHRÛMADHYA (frontal) ★★★

Here, we visualize and realize the circulation of prâna between the nostrils and Bhrûmadhya. This leads to interiorization and deep calm.

Place all your attention on
the inside of the nostrils,
which you consider to be a
subtle center.

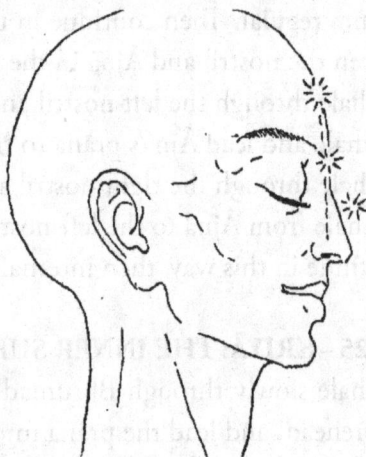

△ Inhale slowly and visualize the subtle breath rising in both nostrils, crossing Trikutî and continuing in a nâdî located slightly under the skin, up to the middle of the forehead at Bhrûmadhya.

▲ Suspend your breath for a moment and center yourself at Bhrûmadhya, mentally looking through this point.

▽ Then exhale and bring the prâna back in the opposite direction, from Bhrûmadhya to the nostrils, crossing Trikutî. With a little practice, you'll be able to feel the entire passage.

Breathing should remain as slow and regular as possible to bring out the subtlety of the mind. But there's nothing to stop you from stopping now and then and letting your natural breathing return, as long as you maintain concentration. In fact, alternating kriyâ with static concentration is highly effective.

Imagination awakens sensation and sensation leads to experience

---

N° 128 – KRIYÂ: NOSTRILS ←→ BRAHMARANDHRA ★★★

Visualize a nâdî between Trikutî and Brahmarandhrafollowing the curve of the forehead and skull.

△ Inhale the prâna through the nostrils and let it rise to the top of the skull, crossing Trikutî, Bhrûmadhya, and following the median line of the forehead and skull.

▽ As you exhale, return from Brahmarandhra to the nostrils.

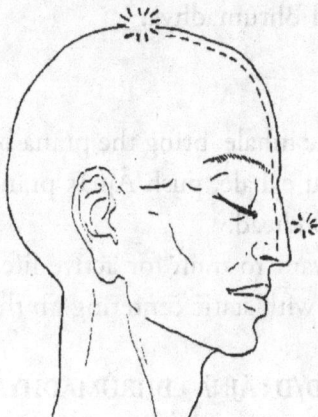

This constitutes a cycle.

Gradually perform several series of 12 cycles, interspersed with static concentration on inner vigilance.

N° 129 – R.D.: THE WITNESS AND THE DISTANT FRONT SPACE ★★★

In the inner space, focus on the position of the witness, detached, observing without reacting to the information he receives. He is the beholder. Position yourself as a witness at Âjnâ chakra. This may take several minutes. Once you've mastered this, start the kriyâ:

△ Inhale: focus on the tell-tale, moving it backwards.

▽ Exhale: focus on the frontal space you are moving away from.
△ Inhale: keep scanning the frontal space.
▽ Exhale: return to the control towards the back of the head.
Perform ten or more cycles. Finish with a static concentration in the control position.

N° 130 – KRIYÂ : ÂJNÂ ←→ BHRÛMADHYA ★★★

Walk the subtle passage
between Bhrûma-dhya and
Âjnâ.
  Concentrate on the
horizontal nâdî between
Âjnâ and Bhrûmadhya.

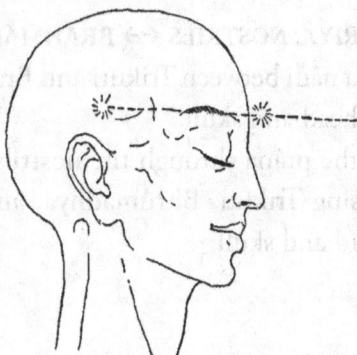

△ On the inhale, bring the prâna back to Âjnâ.
▽ As you exhale, push Âjnâ's prâna towards Bhrûmadhya and beyond
   the forehead.
If you want to train for active life, keep your eyes open. You can also
continue with static centering on the horizontal axis.

N° 131 – D/D : ÂJNÂ + BHRÛMADHYA ★★★
△ Inhale with centering at Bhrûmadhya, in the middle of the forehead.
▽△ Exhale / inhale: centering in Âjnâ.
▽ Exhale and return to Bhrûmadhya.
Balance the left and right sides.

N° 132 – VARIANT, THE AUM VIBRATION IN THE FOREHEAD ★★★
Imagine a flower like the Lily or the Bindweed, with its heart at Âjnâ
and its corolla at forehead level.
△ Inhale regularly, evenly, remaining centered in Âjnâ.
▽ As you exhale, move towards Bhrûmadhya, visualizing the opening of
   the corolla or an energetic expansion at the forehead.

▼ A short empty suspension to prolong your concentration.

VARIANT: THE VIBRATION OF AUM IN THE FOREHEAD ★★★
△ Inspiration: concentration in Âjnâ.
▽ Exhalation: the AUM vibrates from Âjnâ to Bhrûmadhya and then over the whole forehead.
▼ In the shunyaka, prolong your concentration.

N° 133 – KRIYÂ: RELAXATION OF THE BACK OF THE HEAD ★★★
△ At inspiration, lead the prâna from Bhrûmadhya to Âjnâ.
▽ As you exhale, sound the AUM from Âjnâ over the whole of the outer posterior area of the skull, reaching around the ears and around the center of the neck, then over the whole neck to the shoulders. Practice a minimum of ten cycles.

N° 134 – KRIYÂ: THE OPENING OF BRAHMARANDHRA'S COROLLA ★★★
△ Inhale regularly, evenly, remaining centered in Âjnâ.
▽ As you exhale, raise the prâna towards the top of the skull, Brahmarandhra, while visualizing the opening of the corolla or a vibratory expansion at the top of the skull.
▼ Small vacuum suspension concentration.

N° 135 – KRIYÂ: SILENCE ★★★
In the kriyâs of this series, you can achieve exceptional relaxation, or enter states of meditation.

Practice quietly, and look for subtlety in the sensations.
Here, the prânava AUM, is associated with inhalation and exhalation.
△ As you inhale, lead the subtle breath with the sound of the vowels, from the nostrils to Trikutî.

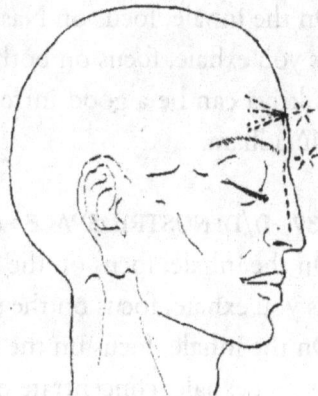

▽ Exhaling as slowly as possible, vibrate the nasal sound along the path from Trikutî to Brûmadhya, then enter the inner space of the head and spread this vibration throughout Chidâkâsh.

Continue this movement for 12 cycles, then listen to the vibration as it continues on its own, leading us to inner silence.

> *Always end your kriyâ with static concentration to assimilate and intensify the effects.*
> *You can consider kriyâ:*
> ◆ *As a support for your attention,*
> ◆ *Like a preparation for still concentration and inner silence.*
> ◆ *An authentic doorway to inner experience.*

The vibration of prâna in the heart

Make sure you've mastered the exercises in Chapter 11, Introduction to subtlety.

(N° 71) – BEE BREATHING AND SOUND IN THE HEART SPACE ★★★

Practice the Bee Breath, Bhrâmarî. When you're fully immersed in the power of sound, concentrate in the chest and let the sound resonate throughout this space.

N° 136 – D/D: NOSTRIL EXPANSION + NASIKÂGRA MUDRÂ ★★★

△ On the inhale, focus on both nostrils and expand them.

▽ As you exhale, focus on the center of the tip of the nose, Nasikâgra.

△ On the inhale, focus on Nasikâgra.

▽ As you exhale, focus on both nostrils and their expansion.

This kriyâ can be a good introduction to a meditation on the heart or on Mûlâdhâra.

N° 137 – D/D: NOSTRIL SPACE + CHEST SPACE ★★★

△ On the inhale, focus on the space between the nostrils.

▽ As you exhale, focus on the space in your chest.

△ On the inhale, focus on the chest area.

▽ As you exhale, concentrate on the space between the nostrils.

You can add the AUM vibration to the exhalation.

N° 138 – KRIYÂ: NOSTRILS ←→ CHEST SPACE ★★★

Breathe evenly and regularly.

△ Inhale slowly, moving the prâna from the nostrils to the throat, tra-
chea and chest space.

▲ Small suspension and short concentration in the chest area.

▽ As you exhale, take the prâna in the opposite direction, from the chest
to the nostrils.

▼ Small suspension with short centering in the nostril space.

N° 139 – KRIYÂ: THE FRONTAL COROLLA ★★★

△ Inhale regularly, remaining centered in the heart chakra, Anâhata.

▲ Short suspension of a few seconds.

▽ As you exhale, visualize the corolla of a flower opening at the front of
the chest.

▼ Prolong concentration with a suspension of breath.

N° 140 – KRIYÂ, THE DOUBLE ELEVATION ★★★

Center yourself in the heart chakra.

△ As you inhale slowly, visualize and feel an upward movement of prâna
through the chakra.

▲ Short suspension of a few seconds.

▽ As you exhale, repeat the same upward movement of the prâna at the
level of Anâhata, in the central channel, Sushumnâ.

The awakening of Sushumnâ and the chakras

N° 141 – KRIYÂ: THE LEMNISCATE ★★★

Concentrate on Sushumnâ, then descend to its base, the Mûlâdhâra
chakra.

Stay at Mûlâdhâra and create a horizontal lemniscate curve with the
center at the chakra. Form 10 lemniscates starting from the left and as
many from the right.

Then raise your center and place yourself at the Swâdhisthâna chakra.
In the same way, form 10 lemniscates starting from the left and 10 lemniscates starting from the right.

Proceed as follows for each chakra: Manipura in the solar plexus, Anâhata in the chest, Vishuddha at the base of the throat, Âjnâ in the head and Brahmarandhra at the top of the skull.

Then practice in the same way, moving down all the chakras. Finish by concentrating on Sushumnâ.

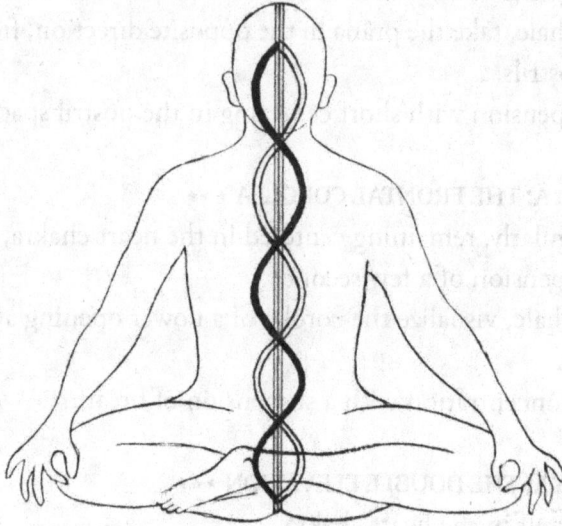

The 3 nâdîs: Sushumnâ, Idâ and Pingalâ

(N° 48) – ASHWINÎ MUDRÂ AND CONCENTRATION IN SUSHUMNÂ ★★★

We have seen the practice of Ashwinî mudrâ. When mastered, increase to 108 contractions/relaxations. In the concentration that follows, concentrate on Sushumnâ. Repeat the whole cycle two or three times.

(N° 86) – PRÂNÂYÂMA WITH THE THREE BANDHAS ★★★

△ Inhale completely, in 5 seconds, for example, and hold for 1 second.

▽ Exhale in 10 seconds.

Then, in order, bend your head and take the Jâlandhara bandha, then press down with your hands on your thighs to realize Uddîyâna bandha, then activate Mûla bandha. These are the three bandhas you'll be holding for the duration of the empty retention.

▼ Keep the breath empty for 15 seconds, closing the glottis tightly, with the three bandhas while concentrating on Sushumnâ. Equalize both hemispheres.

△ At the end of shunyaka, release, in the reverse order in which you took them: Mûla bandha, then Uddîyâna (release the belly), then Jâland-hara (raise the head). Exhale a little to release the breath, then inhale again quietly over 5 seconds.

This forms a cycle. Take a concentration break between each cycle, or link them together without interruption.

Nº 142 – D/D: MÛLÂDHÂRA + SAHASRÂRA ★★★

△ As you inhale, concentrate on Mûlâdhâra.

▽ As you exhale, concentrate on Sahasrâra + *Mûla B.*

△ On the inhale, focus on Sahasrâra.

▽ As you exhale, concentrate on Mûlâdhâra + *Mûla B.*

Practice 10 cycles, then concentrate on Sushumnâ.

Eventually, repeat the same practice two or three times.

Nº 143 – KRIYÂ: MÛLÂDHÂRA ←→ AJNÂ ★★★

Concentrate on Mûlâdhâra. Then visualize the central channel, Sush-umnâ, from Mûlâdhâra to Âjnâ, for a few moments.

Then begin the kriyâ :

△ With inspiration, raise the prâna from Mûlâdhâra to Âjnâ.

▲ Short suspension and concentration in Âjnâ.

▽ As you exhale, bring the prâna down through Sushumnâ to Mûlâd-hâra.

▼ Small suspension with short centering in Mûlâdhâra.

Practice 10 to 12 cycles, then concentrate on Sushumnâ. Eventually, repeat the same practice two or three times.

Nº 144 – KRIYÂ: MÛLÂDHÂRA ←→ SAHASRÂRA ★★★

Concentrate on Mulâdhâra. Then visualize the central channel, Sush-umnâ, from Mûlâdhâra to Sahasrâra, for a few moments.

Then begin the kriyâ :

△ With inspiration, raise the prâna from Mûlâdhâra to Sahasrâra.

▲ Small suspension and centering in Sahasrâra.

▽ As you exhale, bring the prâna back to Mûlâdhâra.

▼ Small suspension and centering in Mûlâdhâra.

Practice 10 cycles, then concentrate on Sushumnâ. Eventually, repeat the same practice two or three times.

N° 145 – KRIYÂ: MÛLÂDHÂRA ←→ SAHASRÂRA IN SQUARE BREATHING
★★★

Concentrate on Mulâdhâra. Then visualize the central channel, Sushumnâ, from Mûlâdhâra to Sahasrâra, for a few moments.

Then begin square breathing, for example 6 : 6 : 6 : 6, in Ujjâyî, with *Khecarî mudrâ*.

△ With inspiration, raise the prâna: from Mûlâdhâra to Sahasrâra.

▲ Suspension for 6 seconds and concentration in Sahasrâra with half a *Mûla bandha*.

▽ On the exhale, bring the prâna back to Mûlâdhâra in 6 seconds.

▼ Suspension of breath with centering in Mûlâdhâra with half a *Mûla bandha*, in 6 seconds.

Practice 10 cycles, then concentrate on Sushumnâ.

Eventually, repeat the same practice two or three times.

APPENDIX:
BUILD YOUR PROGRAM

Three learning stages

We've discovered and experimented with the different elements of a new discipline. But as with any jigsaw puzzle, we need to find a method and organize our progress.

Here is an example of a progression. It's up to you to adapt it more precisely to your own motivation, abilities and objectives.

FIRST STAGE: 2 to 6 months

Build up your session with a possible exercise from each group, respecting the order. The rhythms given correspond to the final objective.

Work on your sitting posture every day

Incorporate full breathing into every session.

Incorporate one exercise from each group as far as possible.

☞ Breathing and bandhas

FIRST GROUP

N° 8 - Abdominal breathing

N° 9 - Complete breathing

N° 24 - Triangular breathing + Kumbhaka with the rhythm 8 : 8 : 8

N° 16 - Relaxing triangular breathing with the 8 : 8 : 8 rhythm

N° 19 - Square breathing, in Ujjâyî, with the Khecari mudrâ

Square breathing (1 : 1 : 1 : 1), rhythm 6 : 6 : 6 : 6

SECOND GROUP

N° 30 - Breathing the four faces: Brahma or Caturmukhi prânâyâma
N° 31 - Clavicular Kâpâlabhâti
N° 29 - Kâpâlabhâti, the bellows 2 series of 108 times

THIRD GROUP

N° 48 - The practice of Ashwinî mudrâ with 2 series of 108 times

FOURTH GROUP

N° 50 - Uddiyâna bandha with 1 series of 3 times

FIFTH GROUP

N° 21 - Alternating breathing, Nâdî Shodana with progressive rhythms 8 : 8 then 7 : 14 then 5 : 10 : 10

SIXTH GROUP

N° 62 - Breathing perfume
N° 63 - Sensations in the nostrils
N° 64 - Expanding nostrils
N° 19 - Ûjjayî prânâyâma
N° 20 - Ujjâyî in Jalandhara bandha
N° 71 - The Breath of the Bee: Bhramari prânâyâma
N° 41 - Shâmbavî, Bhoochari and Agochari mudrâs
N° 42 - Preparing for Shambavi mudrâ

☞ Working on thought and the inner mind

SEVENTH GROUP

♦ Eye relaxation exercises
N° 113 - Bhoochari mudrâ and thoughts
N° 114 - Square breathing and thoughts
N° 115 - D/D: rebalancing brains and thoughts
N° 106 - Palming and interior space
N° 107 - Bhoochari, the mudrâ of emptiness and Chidakash
Variant 2: Empty space

EIGHTH GROUP

N° 95 - The discovery of mental citta
N° 118 - D/D: neck + forehead
N° 119 - D/D: neck + solar plexus
N° 120 - D/D: skull + perineum
N° 121 - Kriyâ: Bhrûmadhya and frontal space
N° 122 - Kriyâ: Anuloma Viloma and Bhrûmadhya) (front)
N° 127 - The nostril path ↔ Bhrûmadhya (frontal)

SECOND STAGE: 2 to 6 months

Build your session with one exercise from each group, respecting the order of the groups. The rhythms given correspond to the final objective. Master the half-lotus or another seated pose.

Incorporate one exercise from each group as far as possible.

☞ **Breathing and bandhas**

FIRST GROUP

N° 57 - Uddiyâna B + Nauli central
N° 53 - Uddiyâna bandha + Jalandhara bandha
N° 54 - Uddiyâna bandha + Mûla bandha
N° 55 - Uddiyâna B + Ashwinî mudrâ.
N° 52 - Agnisâra Dhauti 2 sets of 30 times

SECOND GROUP

N° 29 - Kâpâlabhâti, the bellows 3 series of 108 times
N° 29 - Kapâlabhâti and Bhrûmadhya
N° 97 - Kapâlabhâti and the stability of citta
N° 108 - Kapâlabhâti and frontal space
Variant: the far front space
N° 36 - Bhastrika prânâyâma: 1 series of 108 times

THIRD GROUP

N° 48 - The practice of Ashvini mudrâ 2 series of 108 times
N° 48 - Chapter 13, The practice of ashvini mudrâ and Bhrûmadhya

FOURTH GROUP

N° 50 - Uddiyâna bandha 1 2 series of 3 times

FIFTH GROUP

N° 19 - Square breathing, in Ujjâyî, with the Khecarî mudrâ 8 : 8 : 8 : 8

N° 87 - Square breathing and Bhrûmadhya

N° 22 - Nâdî Shuddhi prânâyâma supérieur, 12 : 6 : 12 : 6

N° 24 - Triangular breathing + Kumbhaka 10 : 10 : 10 + concentration

SIXTH GROUP

N° 21 and 83 - Alternate breathing, Nâdî Shodana with Kumbhaka Rhythm 4 : 16 : 8

SEVENTH GROUP

N° 20 - Ujjâyî in Jalandhara bandha 10 : 10

N° 16 - Triangular relaxation breathing 10 : 10 : 10 + concentration

N° 56 - Prânâyâma triangulaire (Shunyaka) + ½ Uddiyâna bandha 10 : 10 : 10

N° 94 - Prânâyâma triangulaire (Shunyaka) + Mûlâdhâra

EIGHTH GROUP

N° 60 - Sûrya prânâyâma mudrâ (Sâvitrî prânâyâma)

N° 42 - Shambavi mudrâ 2 minutes

N° 104 - Shunyaka and Shâmbavî mudrâ

N° 103 - Square breathing and Shâmbavî mudrâ

N° 98 - Kapâlabhâti, Shâmbavî and Mûla bandhas

☞ Working on thought and the inner mind

NINTH GROUP

N° 43 - Nasikâgra mudrâ and Samatâ prânâyâma: 2 minutes

N° 46 - Akashi mudrâ (citta or ajna)

TENTH GROUP

Continue to train yourself in the observation of thoughts and increase the duration of non-thinking moments.

N° 113 - Bhoochari mudrâ and thoughts

N° 114 - Square breathing and thoughts

N° 115 - D/D: Brain balancing and thoughts

N° 116 - Samatâ prânâyâma and thoughts

ELEVENTH GROUP

In these last two groups, look for subtlety in sensations to induce in the mind a state of deep receptivity and interiorization.

N° 67 - Aum and breathing

N° 72 - Bee breathing: the sound of breathing in and out

Variant – the Bee with concentration

N° 64 - Expanding nostrils

N° 68 - Samatâ prânâyâma and Aum

N° 66 - Samatâ prânâyâma and breath suspension

N° 43 - Nasikâgra mudrâ and Samatâ prânâyâma

N° 75 - The perfect curve

TWELFTH GROUP

N° 121 - Kriyâ: Bhrûmadhya and frontal space

N° 122 - Kriyâ: Anuloma Viloma and Bhrûmadhya) (front)

N° 127 - The nostril path ←→ Bhrûmadhya (frontal)

N° 125 - Kriyâ: the inner surface of the forehead

N° 126 - Kriyâ: Internal skull scanning

N° 129 - D.D.: The witness and the distant frontal space

N° 130 - Kriyâ : Âjnâ ←→ Bhrûmadhya

N° 131 - D/D : Âjnâ + Bhrûmadhya (variant)

THIRD STAGE: 2 to 6 months

Build your session with one exercise from each group, respecting the order of the groups. The rhythms given correspond to the final objective.

Master the half-lotus or another meditation pose. The Lotus is still an ideal that flexible people can strive for.

Incorporate one exercise from each group as far as possible.

☞ **Breathing and bandhas**

FIRST GROUP

N° 48 - The practice of Ashwinî mudrâ 3 series of 108 times

SECOND GROUP

N° 50 - Uddiyâna bandha 1 to 2 series of 3 or more times
N° 51 - Agnisâra Dhauti: 2 sets of 50 times or more
N° 57 - Uddiyâna B + Nauli central: 3 times or more :
Complete nauli: perfect with left and right nauli, then complete. If nauli complete, 2 to 3 series of 20 levogyric rotations, then 2 to 3 dextrogyric series.

THIRD GROUP

N° 29 - Kâpâlabhâti, the bellows 3 series of 108 times
N° 34 - Kâpâlabhâti, chin up
N° 88 - Kapâlabhâti and Âjnâ
N° 110 - Kapâlabhâti and the complete Chidâkâsh
N° 109 - Kapâlabhâti and the upper head space
N° 36 - Bhastrika prânâyâma (abdomen level) 1 series of 108 times

FOURTH GROUP

N° 21 and 83 – Alternating breathing, Nâdî Shodana rhythm 5 : 20 : 10 or more if you intend to use it as a meditation.

FIFTH GROUP

N° 89 - Triangular breathing and Âjnâ
N° 58 - Tribandha + Shunyaka
N° 58 and 94 – Tribandha + Shunyaka + Ajna or Mûlâdhâra
N° 61 - Prâna mudrâ (Shakti, Mûlâdhâra)

☞ **Working on thought and the inner mind**

SIXTH GROUP

N° 42 - Shambavi mudrâ: 3 minutes, or 5 minutes if you intend to use it as a meditation. Once mastered, gradually extend the duration.

N° 93 - Shâmbavî mudrâ and Âjnâ

SEVENTH GROUP

N° 111 - Square breathing + far front and back space

Triangular breathing variation

N° 112 - Square breathing and Chidakash

N° 91 - Samavritti prânâyâma and Âjnâ

EIGHTH GROUP

N° 67 - Aum and breathing

N° 68 - Samatâ prânâyâma and Aum

N° 66 - Samatâ prânâyâma and breath suspension

(No. 43) Ch. 11 – Nasikâgra mudrâ and Samatâ prânâyâma

N° 75 - The perfect curve

N° 76 - Movement in stillness

N° 77 - Inspiration into exhalation and exhalation into inspiration

N° 90 - Samatâ prânâyâma and Âjnâ

N° 136 - D/D: Nostril expansion + Nasikâgra mudrâ

N° 137 - D/D: nostril space + chest space

N° 72 - Bee breathing: the sound of breathing in and out

Variant – the bee with concentration

N° 92 - The prânâyâma of the bee and Âjnâ

N° 72 - The bee and sound in the heart space

☞ **Perfecting the kriyâs, in the spirit of meditation**

NINTH GROUP

N° 123 - Anuloma Viloma: nostrils ←→ Brahmarandhra

N° 124 - Kriyâ: Anuloma Viloma and Âjnâ

N° 125 - Kriyâ: the inner surface of the forehead

N° 126 - Kriyâ: internal skull scanning

N° 127 - The nostril path ←→ Bhrûmadhya (frontal)

N° 128 - Kriyâ: nostrils ←→ Brahmarandhra

N° 129 - D.D.: The witness and the distant frontal space

N° 130 - Kriyâ : Âjnâ ←→ Bhrûmadhya

N° 131 - D/D : Âjnâ + Bhrûmadhya (variant)

N° 132 - Kriyâ: the opening of the âjnâ corolla

Variation: vibration of the Aum in the forehead

N° 133 - Kriyâ: relaxation of the back of the head

N° 134 - The opening of Brahmarandhra's corolla

N° 135 - Kriyâ: silence

N° 136 - kriyâ: nostrils ←→ chest space

N° 139 - Kriyâ: the frontal corolla

N° 140 - Kriyâ: elevation

☞ **The awakening of Sushumnâ and the chakras**

TENTH GROUP

N° 141 - Kriyâ: the lemniscate

N° 54 - The practice of Ashwinî mudrâ and concentration in Sushumnâ

N° 105 - Prânâyâma with the three bandhas

N° 142 - D/D: Mûlâdhâra + Sahasrâra

N° 143 - Kriyâ : Mûlâdhâra ←→ Âjnâ

N° 144 - Kriyâ: Mûlâdhâra ←→ Sahasrâra in square breathing

N° 145 - Kriyâ: Mûlâdhâra ←→ Sahasrâra

FOURTH STAGE

Practices are supposed to be mastered. Then comes the exclusive time for meditation:

In the growth of consciousness-strength (male prâna), with long kumbhakas accompanied by concentration, or with long shunyakas and Uddîyâna bandha with concentrations.

In the subtlety and sensitivity of consciousness (feminine prâna) with subtle breaths, or kriyâs.

In this stage, representations, intentions and concentrations are fundamental.

Build up your session each day, continuing to respect the order of the groups you choose.

Or practice to your heart's content.

HAVE A GOOD PRACTICE!

CONCLUSION:
TRANSCENDENCE THROUGH PRÂNA

The three goals of meditation

We've discovered the pleasure of feminine prâna and the fullness of masculine prâna. They can now serve the three objectives we have assigned to the practice of meditation, which are, let us remember:

◊ Access to transcendence and depth;

◊ Increasing our resources;

◊ Achieving mental silence and thus mastery of thought.

Here we emphasize the possibility that people with strong intellectual energy, who might therefore find it difficult to eliminate thought, can more easily achieve thought control through the perception and practice of prâna.

What can we expect from breathing?

Seated meditation, in the service of deep interiorization and the exclusive growth of consciousness, may be a royal road to cultivating the essential in the human being, but in our time it is no longer the only and imperative path for our spiritual evolution.

Transcendence through prâna

Subtle breathing and kriyâs, along with practices that promote feminine prâna, lead to transcendence through bliss and energy, and connect us to the individual Divine, particularly in the Heart.

The perception and development of prâna, as well as the recognition of force-consciousness, which is cultivated in breath-holding and dynamization bandhas, all go in the same direction towards integrating outer life more fully into our goals of transformation and self-transcendence. In particular, breath-holding, combined with concentration, especially on the prâna, can considerably stimulate our chakras and the consciousness-force of Sushumnâ, which has mainly been used in the quest for liberation, but which is waiting for us to use its transformative power too.

As we've said, Tantra insists on the close relationship between breathing and prâna, between prâna and citta, between citta and the psyche. So, through breathing, we can act and transform our vitality, our emotions and our thoughts, without passing through the filter of morality and will. But breathing can take us even further. For prâna is also a gateway to universal spiritual energy and Psychic Being. In breath-holding and in kriyâs, prâna can become the support of consciousness and promote all kinds of transformations.

We know of nothing better than prânâyâma for increasing and strengthening prâna and our internal energy, and nothing more effective for eliminating depression or increasing concentration and inner strength. Prânâyâma leads us not only to strength and energy, but also to the joy of being.

The techniques associated with prâna bring great satisfaction and happiness. For prâna is linked to energy, enjoyment, power, abundance and fulfillment. And the more we cultivate it, the more we connect with it – and the more remarkable its effects.

> *Awareness, accumulation and subtilization of prâna
> increases all our resources tenfold.*

These practices bring to meditation, the medium of the essential, a little of those two traits that are often lacking in classical meditations: **the bliss** that characterizes the supreme Reality, Existence-Consciousness-Beatitude, in the Indian tradition, and the **Energy** that accompanies this same Reality as soon as it becomes incarnated in material Manifestation.

What are the greatest resources at our disposal?

Breath and the prâna it carries are our first and most available resource. But more precisely, consciousness and its corollary, strength-consciousness, together with prâna, are our most important resources. As we shall see in the next volume.

So many people around the world have developed exceptional abilities in mind, body or spirit. And Nature on Earth is so rich! In the material realm, we have discovered it through scientific research, but also more broadly, through our sensitivity as human beings, and this has enabled the emergence of all the poetry and sensitivity to beauty and higher emotions, which are present in all civilizations.

And if we place ourselves in the field of a more accomplished sensibility, that of the first peoples, that of our sensitives, and of all the yogis of the Earth, we can realize the wonder of our energetic and subtle bodies, or the unlimited potentialities of the multitude of devas and nature spirits.

And yet, in the face of all these marvels and potentialities of Nature, there is such misery, such unconsciousness, such suffering among human beings. What's wrong?

We may think that Higher Nature's objective is to create civilizations and empires, but behind these objectives there is a deeper secret meaning for the soul, which is the development of individual consciousness. It's clear that we're not using the resources at our disposal; we're only operating at 10% of our capacity, it's been said. Why is this? We see two reasons: the first is internal: we don't know or imagine these profound resources. The second is external: humanity is enslaved to forces that monopolize all wealth and fight everything that can lead to individual evolution.

Apart from the military, who is interested in these individual resources[1]? Note that if the military were interested in the growth of the vital force, prâna, it would run the risk of becoming non-violent, because the function of prâna is to create and sustain life, not destroy it! And it's because Prâna and Life are egoless – because they are infinite[2] – that the scientist is unwilling to recognize and study life and consciousness. Otherwise, he'd be obliged to leave behind this persona of

1. In today's world, the military is turning to transhumanism and "augmented man".
2. They can, however, reinforce the ego if the person uses prâna for personal gain.

power and develop humility in the face of the grandeur of Nature and its creative process. The mind, by nature, is arrogant – and all the more so the narrower it is. Yes, the institutionalized scientific mind of our time is narrow. It is infinitely complex, but confined to a narrow bandwidth.

Growing awareness

Readers may be surprised at our questioning of the scientific institution, or rather the instrument of its research, the rational mind, originally conceived as a means of seeking knowledge both legitimately governed by irreproachable logic and in reaction to religious power and its mentality. But you can't develop an irreproachable mentality when you're in reaction (religion) or in conflict of interest (industry). Starting with a methodology adapted to the laboratory and the material field of research, the methodology was then extended to the entire terrestrial sphere of life and mind, and became the spearhead of a Unique Thought where any form of thought different from an exclusively materialistic position had to be fought. Scientific methodology became an ideology, even a dogma. In fact, scientific power simply replaced religious power and hegemony.

On the other hand, Logic – as the ancient thinkers of all great civilizations, and in particular India and Tibet, have demonstrated – must not limit its field of action[1] since its objective is Truth in itself. For the ancient philosophers, thinkers and sages were attached to the idea of Truth and universal Knowledge, an idea today abandoned by modern philosophers enslaved to conforming to the superficial ideas of the age.

This Single Thought, opposed by nature to the growth of individual consciousness and to all human diversity and Nature's biodiversity, proved to be a godsend for the entire commercial and financial sphere, which could extend its power without limits.

For there are two sides to Science: on the one hand, basic research, and on the other, its application in unlimited technology. Fundamental research is hampered by this exclusively sensory ideology – that which cannot be perceived by our gross senses is considered non-existent. As a result, science has decreed that Life and Consciousness cannot exist without a material basis. Technology has thus become a prodigious tool for

1. And therefore not to limit the field of research to the material and sensory plane alone.

reinforcing the power of the economy and finance, and for generalizing censorship of any **technological alternative** that would promote individual autonomy or a collective good that would threaten the interests of merchants and elites, but also for censoring all the diversity of ideological, philosophical and spiritual alternative thought.

A dictatorship has already taken hold across the globe. The example of China, but also to a lesser extent Europe, in the surveillance of the masses by spyware hidden throughout the IT sphere, and in the manipulation of information mainly by the media corrupted by their billionaire owners, shows us clearly that this is the case.

Two questions emerge from this observation. The first is: "What is the future of diversity in humanity and in the Nature that nurtures and surrounds it, and in particular the freedom to think, and what is therefore the future of philosophy and spirituality?"

The second question is"What can we do?"

And that's when we realize that our awareness is urgent and becoming imperative, and that the only solution left to counterbalance this powerful hegemony and emerging global dictatorship is **the growth of individual consciousness, and its corollary, inner strength**, not to escape earthly reality, but to fulfill the human and life.

The human being is a formidable free-energy machine

We need to differentiate between Surunity and Free Energy. Surunity is an alternative technical concept that postulates a technology based not on entropy, but on negentropy. In other words, the energy of a motor, for example, is greater at its output. If we introduce 1 joule at the input, we have 1.5 joules at the output. Numerous researchers have produced such devices. Free Energy, on the other hand, is unlimited access to the energy of the universe – also known as zero-point energy – and concerns all areas of life on earth and in Nature, not only technology, but also intelligence, education or personal development, the arts, philosophy, health or politics.

Free Energy is the universal creative energy. We believe that in the next ten to twenty years, it will gradually replace all the energy sources we know in our predatory civilization for ourselves and our environment.

This unlimited conscious energy will be used in all fields and will reshape all parts of our consciousness and nature. Whether science and spirituality, agriculture and medicine, architecture, education or interplanetary travel, everything will be unified in an unlimited evolutionary curve.

As human beings, our egotic consciousness means that we operate in a vacuum, looping around in the system, in our mind, our life force and in the life of the body. That's why we're so stressed, so weak in the face of adversity, so selfish and egocentric, so exposed to suffering, so subject to disease. And our technology, our philosophy, our social life and our individual condition all reflect this.

In this closed circuit, the vision of science bears a great responsibility for having closed all the doors of Nature and Matter, right down to the infinitely small, by filling in all the instabilities, all the[1] voids, all the gaps, in a frenzied multiplication of rational reference points to eliminate everything it couldn't understand or control and which it baptized error, artifact, chance, charlatanism or esotericism. We are condemned to devour our environment, sterilize our surroundings and dry up our planet, because we are poisoning ourselves and we have less and less means of regenerating ourselves, since we have cut ourselves off from Mother Nature, who holds all the keys to energy and consciousness.

In the image of medicine, which has turned the body into a sick fortress, enslaved to the chemical drugs it sells at high prices, and the Genetic Vaccine, an obligatory poison renamed the savior of humanity, which will reshape us and correct Nature's errors in our DNA, in the image of our religions, our philosophies and our politics, which have confined all possibilities to a vision and a situation of dependence and enslavement, all our horizons are systematically blocked or dangerously threatened.

And as long as we refuse to recognize that life and consciousness can only function through exchange, as long as we are unable to conceive of an alliance between unity and multiplicity, and as long as we cannot accept that we can be governed and nourished by a universal consciousness and energy, the situation will worsen and Nature will lead us into painful impasses.

1. Today's cutting-edge quantum physics tells us, on the contrary, that the vacuum is the richest medium and conceals unlimited energy. In fact, the vacuum between the particles of matter is at least 99.9999% of the amount of matter in the universe.

And yet the superior Nature that fashioned us has endowed us with numerous channels, all more fundamental than the others, to connect us to this unlimited universal energy and all its worlds, for knowledge, fullness of life, joy and abundance, health and immortality. But we have polluted or condemned all these doors, all these passages. We've closed everything off and locked ourselves into this individual and collective system we've created. Perhaps this was necessary or inevitable in the context of this planetary experiment. We're not going to apply any morality to it.

Prâna is one of these passages through the Manipura chakra and the Hara. Let's prepare for its blossoming with the disciplines and exercises described in this book.

Another world—of Light—may be just around the corner, but to get there we'll have to cross the swamp. May the power of Light be with us!

INDEX OF SANSKRIT WORDS
AND SPECIFIC TERMS

A

Bee (prânâyâma de l'), N°71

Agnisâra dhauti, N°52

Âjnâ chakra, the inner mind center in the head

Âkâshi mudrâ, N°46

Anâhata chakra: the Heart chakra.

Ânanda: bliss or spiritual joy.

Anuloma viloma: psychic alternate breathing.

Apâna vâyu, the prâna in the body whose function is elimination

Âsanas: yoga postures

Âshram: monastic community in India

Ashvinî mudrâ, N°48

Âtman: the Divine in its universal form

Âyâma: extension, growth

B

Bandha: muscular contraction influencing psyche and prâna

Bhastrikâ prânâyâma: breathing in the same family as Kapâlabhâti, Le Soufflet, No. 29

Bhoochari mudrâ, N°39

Bhrâmarî prânâyâma: the Bee, N°70

Bhrûmadhya: the subtle center in the middle of the forehead, see table ch. 11

Buddhi: the intellectual and superior mind

Brahman: the Divine

Brahmarandhra: the frontal projection of the Sahasrâra chakra at the top of the skull

C

Chaïtya purusha: the Psychic Being, chapter 2

Chakra: energy center of the subtle body

Chidâkâsh: the inner space of the head, chapter 15

Chit: consciousness

Chit-Shakti or Chit-Tapas: consciousness-strength or consciousness-energy

Chitta or citta: substance of consciousness, chapter 14.

D

Dhâranâ: a stage of meditation, uninterrupted concentration or contemplation

Dhyâna: meditation

Dynamic Duality: chapter 17

E

Inner space: see Chidâkâsh chapter 15.

Psychic Being: chapter 2

Hatha yoga: body yoga

I

Idâ: one of the 3 main energy channels, table in chapter 8.

J

Jâla, network, net

Jâlandhara bandha: throat contraction, No. 80

jivanmukta: liberated yogi, having attained spiritual realization and the end of the Wheel of Births

Jivâtma or Jivâtman: the individual Divine, chapter 2

Jnâna: knowledge

K

Kali yuga: the iron age

Kapâlabhâti prânâyâma, Le Soufflet, N° 29

Khecarî mudrâ, N° 40

Kosha: body, envelope

Kriyâ: tantric energy technique chapter 17

Kshetram: front part of a chakra

Kumbhaka: breath-holding with full lungs

Kundalinî shakti: the individual Divine in the form of energy, the individual Consciousness-Force. Kundalinî is to energy what the Psychic Being is to consciousness.

M

Mahâbhastrikâ: the great Bhastrikâ

Maha bandha or **Tribandha:** the 3 bandhas Jâlandhara, Uddîyâna and Mûla

Mâlâ: Indian rosary

Manas: sensory, lower mind and, by extension, ordinary mind

Manipûra chakra, the belly chakra, center of dynamic vitality

Mantra: sound or set of sounds influential in yoga

Mâyâ: illusion

Mâyâ: the cosmic illusion

Mudrâ (fem)**:** gesture or body position influencing the psyche and prâna

Mukha: head, face

Mûla bandha: contraction of the sphincters of the anus, N° 47

Mûlâdhâra chakra: the base chakra

Muni mudrâ, N° 37

N

Nâdî: energy channel in the subtle physical body

Nâdî shodana: alternate breathing, No. 21

Nasikâgra mudrâ: concentrating the gaze on the tip of the nose

O

Upanishad: Indian spiritual texts after the Vedas

P

Padmâsana: the Lotus posture, illustration chapter 4

Pingalâ: one of the 3 main energy channels, table in chapter 8

Plavini prânâyâma, one of the prânâyâmas specific to Hatha-Yoga, enabling you to float on water.

Prakriti: Universal Nature

Prâna: internal energy, vital force or universal energy

Prânamaya kosha: the energy body, which also includes the vital body

Prânâyâma: the science of yogic breathing

Prânava: the AUM mantra

Pratyâhâra, interiorization, one of the stages of meditation

Pourousha or Purusha: Conscious Being, chapter 2.

R

Râjas: principle of action and reaction

Rectangular breathing: see Sâvitrî prânâyâma, No. 25

Rishis: yogis, sages, seers of the Vedic era

S

Sadhak: disciple following a spiritual path

Sâdhanâ: yogic or spiritual discipline

Sahasrâra chakra: the center above the skull, the Lotus of a thousand petals,

Samâdhi: spiritual trance

Samâna vâyu, the prâna responsible for assimilation

Samatâ prânâyâma: slow, regular, subtle breathing, with equalized duration of inhalation and exhalation, N°65

Samavritti prânâyâma: square breathing, No. 26

Sâmkhya: one of India's philosophical systems

Sâvitrî prânâyâma, rectangular breathing, N°25

Shakti: the energy and force of the Divine, or individual strength-consciousness

Shâmbavî mudrâ, N°42

Sherpa prânâyâma, No. 27

Shiva: the pure consciousness aspect of the Divine

Shunyaka: breath-holding with empty lungs

Siddhâsana: a seated yoga posture, table chapter 4

Subliminal: the subliminal nature is the deep and luminous mental, vital and physical nature.

Supraconscious: everything that transcends individual consciousness

Supramental: world or Gnostic consciousness beyond the universal mind

Sûrya: sun

Sûrya Bhedana, one of the specific breaths of Hatha Yoga

Sushumnâ: one of the 3 main energy channels, table in chapter 8

Swâddhisthâna chakra, the chakra of the abdomen, linked to Vital Sensory and the water element

T

Tamas: principle of inertia, one of the three gunas.

Tantra: Tantrism

Tantras: traditional Tantric scriptures,

Trikutî: energy center of the head, table chapter 11

U

Udâna vâyu, see the 5 prânas, table chapter 8

Uddîyâna bandha: withdrawing from the belly with empty lungs. N° 50

Ujjâyî prânâyâma, N° 19

Ûrdhva, upwards

V

Vâyu, subtle energy in the body

Vedas: India's first traditional spiritual scriptures

Vedânta: Indian spiritual philosophy

Vishuddha or **Vishuddhi chakra:** the throat chakra, responsible for expression and the sensory mind, Manas

Vyâna vâyu, see the 5 prânas, table chapter 8

Y

Yama, control, mastery

Yoga nidrâ: deep relaxation, conscious "sleep practice

EXERCISE INDEX

(N° 46) - Akashi mudrâ ★★★

Chapter 15: introduction to interior space
The inner space, Chidâkash
N° 106 - Inner space with palming ★★★
N° 107 - Bhoochari, the mudrâ of emptiness and Chidakash ★★★
N° 108 - Kapâlabhâti and frontal space
Variant : The far front space
N° 109 - Kapâlabhâti and the upper head space
N° 110 - Chidâkâsh complete after Kapâlabhâti ★★★
N° 111 - Square breathing + far front and back space
Triangular breathing variant
N° 112 - Chidakash with square breathing ★★★

Chapter 16: Introduction to thought control
N° 113 - Bhoochari mudrâ and thoughts ★★★
N° 114 - Square breathing and thoughts ★★★
N° 115 - Brain balancing and thoughts ★★★
N° 116 - Samatâ prânâyâma and thoughts ★★★
N° 117 - Sâvitrî prânâyâma and self-awareness ★★★

Chapter 17: Introduction to kriyâs
Some rebalancing
N° 118 - D/D: neck / forehead
N° 119 - D/D: neck / solar plexus
N° 120 - D/D: skull + perineum
The deep mind and inner vigilance
N° 121 - Kriyâ: Bhrûmadhya and frontal space ★★★
N° 122 - Kriyâ: nostrils ←→ Bhrûmadhya (Anuloma Viloma) (frontal) ★★★
N° 123 - Kriyâ: Anuloma Viloma: nostrils ←→ Brahmarandhra (frontal)★★★
N° 124 - Kriyâ: Anuloma Viloma and Âjnâ ★★★
N° 125 - Kriyâ: the inner surface of the forehead
N° 126 - Kriyâ: internal skull scanning ★★★

If you would like to be kept informed of our courses
and workshops, or if you would like to organize one,
please contact the author at his email address:

patrice@savitri.fr

In 1969, Patrice Godart interrupted his training as a professional airplane pilot to set off on the roads of India. He discovered spiritual yoga in 1970 with La Mère at Sri Aurobindo's ashram in Pondicherry. He stayed there for over a year, returning regularly.

He met Baba Muktananda on several occasions and learned yoga at various centers and ashrams, in Bénarés, Rameshwaram, Rishikesh, at the Lonavla Yogic Hospital, with Pattaby Joïs in Mysore, but above all at Paramahansa Satyananda's ashram in Monghyr. In his early years of contact with India, he repeatedly experienced the powerful antagonistic realizations of worldly illusion and individual Divinity.

From 1977 onwards, he embarked on a two-pronged approach: on the one hand, the study and experimentation of the influence of Form and sacred architecture, as part of a multidisciplinary team; and on the other, a sustained practice of yoga (hatha, prânâyâma, yoga nidrâ, kriyâ yoga) and its teaching. This has led him to discover new keys to further integrating the fulfillment of human nature and the liberation of consciousness.

He thus advocates a multiple, progressive and diversified practice in the inner life, and insists on the necessary balance between spiritual realization, the transformation of human nature, and the outer life, that of everyone's daily life.

Fifty years of reflection, personal experience and teaching have prompted him to share the fruits of his experience.

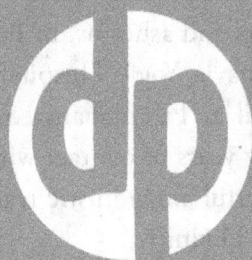

Discovery Publisher is a multimedia publisher
whose mission is to inspire and support personal
transformation, spiritual growth and awakening.
We strive with every title to preserve the essential
wisdom of the author, spiritual teacher, thinker,
healer, and visionary artist.

www.ingramcontent.com/pod-product-compliance
Lightning Source LLC
Chambersburg PA
CBHW011223300326
41935CB00044BA/1798

* 9 7 8 1 7 8 8 9 4 6 3 9 1 *